T0115253

CODE RED FALLUJAH

Advance Praise for *Code Red Fallujah*

"In the summer of 2008, while on a USO tour in Iraq to visit our troops, I met Lieutenant Commander Donnelly Wilkes. He was serving as a doctor with the US Navy supporting US Marines stationed in Al Qa'im near the Syrian border. This was his second deployment. His first in was in 2004, attached to the 1st Marine Division during the Battle of Fallujah. In our conversation at Al-Qa'im, it turned out we lived in the same area in California and years later we would bump into each other at a local restaurant. That night he reminded me that we had met in Iraq and I thanked him for serving in the Navy. Now he has written *Code Red Fallujah*, a memoir of his days in the service, centering on one of the most violent battles of the Iraq war—the first of two battles for Fallujah. His faith is tested, his skills as a physician are tested, his family is tested, and his love for the Marines he served with is clear and deep and 'Always Faithful.' A powerful story based on his diaries from the front, I am thankful to support this wonderful book and applaud him for telling his story."

> — Gary Sinise, Actor, Author of *Grateful American,*
> and Founder, Gary Sinise Foundation

"Stripped bare of veneer, out of the toughest fighting in Iraq, comes this moving narrative of a Navy doctor caught up in the battle of Fallujah. Assigned to a front-line Marine infantry battalion, Wilkes's account reveals the human side of being tested by the rigors of war. Read this to understand the sacrifices of America's warriors when called to stand and deliver."

> — General Jim Mattis, U.S. Marines (ret.)
> and 26th Secretary of Defense

"I was a teenager during the time of the Vietnam conflict, and only due to the fact that I had a high draft number during the lottery back then did I escape the all too real possibility that I would have ended up involved in that conflict. The awareness of that is largely responsible for why I am involved with veteran causes to the extent I am, which includes nineteen years hosting the National Memorial Day Concert in our nation's capital. I do this to honor the heroics of the men and women throughout our nation's history who have taken it upon themselves to serve our country, regardless of sacrifice to life and limb. Dr. Donnelly Wilkes is one such individual, and *Code Red Fallujah* is a vivid recount of what the sacrifices are that our men and women of the military have made and continue to make on our behalf. The recount of his experiences during this country's conflict in the Middle East is a powerful reminder of how much we owe to those who have taken on the task as defenders of not just our country, but the hopes and dreams of freedom-loving people everywhere."

— Joe Mantegna, Actor

"As a twenty-three-year Marine Corps veteran, I'm proud to endorse this work. *Code Red Fallujah* transports you back to a time when so many Americans, still reeling from the aftermath of 9/11, felt the call to action— to take on something larger than themselves. As this book unfolds, you'll experience the adventure and chaos Lieutenant Wilkes and his battalion faced in Fallujah. Intertwined with combat action, spiritual challenges, and medical drama—*Code Red Fallujah* is a must read. Dr. Wilkes is still taking care of Marines today…me specifically…he's my doctor! 'Thanks Doc!'"

— Rob Riggle, Marine, Actor, and Comedian

CODE RED FALLUJAH

A DOCTOR'S MEMOIR AT WAR

DONNELLY WILKES, M.D.

A POST HILL PRESS BOOK
ISBN: 978-1-64293-802-9
ISBN (eBook): 978-1-64293-803-6

Code Red Fallujah:
A Doctor's Memoir at War
© 2021 by Donnelly Wilkes, M.D.
All Rights Reserved

Cover art by Cody Corcoran

All people, locations, events, and situations are portrayed to the best of the author's memory. While all of the events described are true, many names and identifying details have been changed to protect the privacy of the people involved.

No part of this book may be reproduced, stored in a retrieval system, or transmitted by any means without the written permission of the author and publisher.

Post Hill Press
New York • Nashville
posthillpress.com

Published in the United States of America
1 2 3 4 5 6 7 8 9 10

To my wife Katie:
They say being a military wife can be the toughest job of all —
you made it look easy. Thank you for your personal sacrifice, and
devotion. Through your love and God's grace, this work has come to life.

To my family Mike and Jan; Riley, John, Michael, Brady, Jennifer:
I'm so blessed to have you in my life. Your unwavering faith
has helped me endure the storms of life. I love you all.

To the men, families, and the lost of 1st Battalion, 5th Marines OIFII:
You are the fabric of the red, white, and blue!
You are in my heart forever.

CONTENTS

CHAPTER 1

Origins,
Sept 11th, 2001

NEW ORLEANS, SEPT 11TH, 2001

The alarm sounds sharply at 5:30 a.m. My hand instinctively pounds the snooze button. I'm slow to rise, but my spirits lift quickly thinking about my sunrise run down St. Charles Avenue, just a few blocks from my apartment in Uptown New Orleans. Patient rounds start at Charity Hospital at 9:00 a.m. sharp, and I have much to do before then: check in on patients, gather overnight data, and prepare my notes. I'm always sharper if I can get a run in beforehand. I'm in my fourth year at Tulane University School of Medicine and sixth year living in New Orleans, the city that has become my second home and truly a source of love in my life. Six years ago, I left my life in California and drove with my father and youngest brother Brady to a foreign world: New Orleans, Louisiana.

My pursuit to become a physician is in full swing; years of education and relentless applications have paid off and nothing can stop me. The city consumes me with its mystical beauty, blended cultures, exotic southern foods, and historical roots. Medicine has a deep history here, dating back to the seventeen hundreds, and the city boasts one of the oldest hospitals in America. I soak it up, every class, every textbook, and the wise professors' words that lay heavy on my ears. Endless hours of study and late nights on call give me the confidence to stay on top, all of it inching me towards my dream of becoming a medical doctor.

In my spare time I am an explorer of foods, culture, and territory. I'm on my adventure and I love it. I live in three different parts of the city, work at three different restaurants, and eat things I've never heard of: turtle soup, alligator boudin, and crawfish étouffée. I explore and photograph my travels, often by myself, walking the French Quarter and driving along the bayous. I go to a cemetery, walk among aboveground tombstones, and meet a voodoo queen. After waiting tables at midnight, I hop a Mississippi paddle boat, play poker with my tip money, and drink old-fashioneds with locals until dawn. On Sunday I walk the inner city, duck into an all-black church and sing hymns as best I can. I walk the Garden District and along the levee, taking photographs as my witness—one of them sells for one hundred dollars at a coffee shop. I wade in water up to my knees during Hurricane Mitch, dance in the end zone at the Louisiana Superdome, and get held up at gunpoint on St. Charles Avenue, escaping unscathed. I deliver a baby in the Louisiana boondocks, escort a southern princess to a debutante ball, and walk eight miles in a crawfish suit at a Mardi Gras parade. I never hesitate or question my place; it is where I am supposed to be.

Finally, I'm a breath away from my medical degree, finishing my final rotations as a fourth-year medical student. Life is good. The Navy granted me a full scholarship to pay for medical school and

I am selected for my choice of residency at Naval Hospital Camp Pendleton upon graduation. In return, I owe them seven years of active duty service. In peacetime, this will involve three years working at a naval hospital, followed by four years of active duty service. My active duty time will either be stateside with the Marines or on a Navy ship in the Pacific. In both cases, I will likely only deploy for seven to ten months—an easy commitment by military standards. During the summer breaks, I attend field medical school and officer training in Newport, Rhode Island; it's the Navy's version of boot camp for officers, preparing me to be a Naval officer and an expert in combat medicine.

On a trip home in August I meet Katie Kogler, the girl I've been looking for. My parents host an annual fifties swing dance in our hometown, Placerville, California. Katie's father Tim plays guitar in the band and is a close friend of my parents. I've known him since I was a child. This year, Tim decides to bring his family from southern California to the dance; he has four daughters I've never met. Katie and I connect immediately; she is twenty-one, with long dark brown hair, blue eyes, fair skin, and a smile that lights up the room. We dance the night away in the warm August summer night. I tell her I'm nearly a doctor and an officer in the Navy, she wrinkles her nose, laughs and asks to see my peacoat! The weekend ends with high hopes and I head back to New Orleans. Over the next few weeks, we talk nearly every night, sharing stories of our lives, mine in medical school, hers finishing college at UCLA. Her father has just been diagnosed with lung cancer. He is the center of her life and the news is heartbreaking, but she is hopeful as he enters treatment. We make plans for her to come to New Orleans for Mardi Gras and I can't wait to show her my world.

Without haste, my shoes are laced up and I'm out the door. It's comfortably warm at seventy-eight degrees; a light green gecko side steps on the wall as I skip down the white porch. Turning down the alley, I smell fresh fall scents, dew mixed with oak leaves permeates the air. I pick up the pace, crossing Canal Street, heading southeast towards the Mississippi River. The uptown area is dense with houses, mostly older shotgun style, usually no more than twelve feet wide, with doors at each end and front porches with ceiling fans and wrought-iron gates, many of them renovated to maintain southern appeal. The larger homes have columns, high doors with wooden sashes, and gas lamps flickering at all hours. In a few blocks, I make the turn onto St. Charles Avenue, sprinting onto the grassy center divider. I run parallel to the trolley tracks, and looking ahead, I see the trolley cars already hard at work. They stop every few blocks to load and unload early risers and drop off patrons to the coffee shops already busy serving customers. As I run downtown, the sun creeps up over the city, gently begging mist to rise from the tracks. I take deeper breaths as my legs move faster and I gain speed along St. Charles Avenue, moving deeper into the garden district of the city. The homes become more palatial with every block. Creole townhouses boast luscious courtyards, thick stone walls, arcades, and cast iron balconies that suggest their strong French and Spanish influence. Tropical ferns and palms border the sidewalks, neatly trimmed red roses surround wraparound white porches—every detail is carefully attended to.

I'm at full speed now, chest heaving with every stride, sweat spilling from my brow. I want to keep going, striding right into downtown and deep into the French Quarter, catching the sweet smell of fresh beignets on Royal Street, or the hearty aroma of chicory coffee in Jackson Square, but my watch tells me it's time to turn around. I slow to a comfortable pace, then to a walk, and before turning back, I stop to look around, standing right on the trolley tracks. Giant oaks with branches like spider legs stretch over my head and sunrays speckle my face through the leaves as a light breeze cools my face. My mind is at ease, my heart is full, I'm right where I want to be.

Once I'm home, it's a rush to get showered, dressed, and out the door. I'm in the middle of my surgical rotation, so green scrubs are a quick and welcome uniform of the day. It's 6:30 a.m. and I'm running behind; breakfast will have to be a protein bar and coffee. I grab my white coat and I'm finally out the door. It's a short white coat, the kind all medical students are given on day one of their first year. I take pride in knowing its days are numbered, as I'll trade it in for a long white coat upon graduation. I jump in my beat up two-door sedan, swallow a gulp from my coffee mug, and throttle towards Canal Street. I go over my patients in my head; I need to check on them before rounds begin with my attending physician. I plan my route through the post-surgical ward of Tulane's hospital, first checking on new lab results, then nursing reports, vital signs, and overnight events.

Finally, I'll enter the room of each patient to examine them and address any concerns. I'll make notes as I go, carefully entering each detail on my template, all designed to provide a snapshot of each person's status for the attending doctor.

I arrive downtown in good time. The closest parking is a grassy lot under a freeway overpass, where I tip the attendant a few dollars and hustle towards the medical school. Tulane's Medical School is one of the oldest in the country. The school was founded in 1834 as the Medical College of Louisiana, the fifteenth oldest in the U.S. and second oldest in the deep south. The school is linked by a walkway to three hospitals, Tulane University Hospital, Veterans Affairs Hospital, and Charity Hospital, giving students excellent hands-on clinical experience and medical training. Charity Hospital was founded in 1736 by a grant from Jean Louis, a French sailor, and is the second oldest continuously operated public hospital in the United States. Those halls are rich with history and tradition, and training in that hallowed place fueled my love for medicine and gave me appreciation for the adventure it is to live in New Orleans. Entering the hospital, I see the clock reads 7:30 a.m. I flash my ID badge to the receptionist, offer a rushed half-smile and "good morning," and head right for the stairs. I have one hour to complete my work and make rounds on time. My data collection goes smoothly, nurses are nice, lab results are ready on time, and my patients are in good spirits without any reported overnight events. It's 8:45 a.m. I'm right on time. Notes in hand and stethoscope tucked into my white coat pocket, I head back to the third-floor walkway from Charity to the medical school. Exiting the double doors onto the breezy walkway, I see friends on the street below hustling into the school, but I wave and keep moving.

As I near the end of the walkway, I see a large group of people on the other side of the glass double doors. They're gathered in a half-circle staring at a television mounted on the wall, a common pit stop for coffee and conversation before class. The group seems excessively large, so I slow down to glance at the TV. Smoke rises from two buildings as headlines flash "Both twin towers hit by planes, possible terrorist attack." Only now do I see the distress on others' faces and recognize the gravity of what is happening. The United States has been attacked! I'm astonished at the sight of the burning buildings, bewildered at how such a thing could happen to us. A feeling of dread comes over me as I stare at sobbing, terrified New Yorkers running through ashen streets. My sadness quickly turns to anger, and all I can think of is "Oh God, what can we do now, what happens next?"

Amidst the commotion, I remember I still have to meet for rounds, and as I walk through the halls everyone is talking, sharing details of the tragedy as it unfolds. The rest of the day is somber, all of us realizing that the world is witnessing an unprecedented event, one that will reshape our lives. I have the sense that my Navy commitment will change, transforming from peacetime to wartime. That night Katie and I talk on the phone, about the incomprehensible number of deaths and fears for our future. I share with her my sadness over the level of hatred in the world and frustration about what to do about it. I tell her my life will change. I'm still six months from graduation and active duty, so I'm not sure exactly how, but I tell her momentum has shifted, and so will my life as a Naval officer.

Graduation comes quickly in July 2002. My whole family comes out for the occasion; it's the first time they have all been together with me in New Orleans. In order of birth, we are Riley, Donnelly, John, Michael, and Brady, with ten years of difference between the oldest and the youngest. Riley and I are identical twins, sharing a parallel life since day one; like many twins we have a special bond. On challenging days, we battle it out to no end, seeking only to best the other, but always find our common blood will surmount any ill will and our friendship as brothers will see us through the most difficult parts of our lives.

My father is Michael Richard Wilkes. He is a self-trained carpenter, and a sheriff as his second career. He grew up in the San Fernando Valley of southern California, moving to our home in northern California after marrying my mother Janet Louise Zemba. He pre-

ferred to spend the weekends coaching his boys in baseball and tend-
ing to our five acres.

Conservative, loving, and patriotic, he was everything I wanted
to be. He was demanding and hardworking to a fault, and I vowed
to take my education as far as I could go, which took me away from
the type of work he loved as a carpenter. My dad taught me to shake
a man's hand and look him in the eye, and that honesty is paramount.
It is him I looked up to and mirrored as I grew into manhood.

My mother, on the other hand, possessed that subtle combination
of kindness, humor, and wit that sanded my rough edges smooth. She
calmed my senses and showed me the tender sides of life. Her voice
mellowed my pains and fears when circumstances seemed their worst,
and her kindness showed me the meaning of empathy towards others.
She helped me trust in myself and the paths I chose in my life.

We are a family with military and law enforcement origins. My
grandfather, Lieutenant John Richard Wilkes, was a World War II
P-38 fighter pilot. He was shot down by the Germans in North
Africa and he survived and went on to serve in the Korean War. He
married my grandmother Kathleen Donnelly and was part of what
Tom Brokaw has coined "The Greatest Generation." In all my mem-
ories, their patriotism was unfailing, through triumph and tragedy;
America was their home team with steadfast devotion. They lived just
down the street from us for most of my life. My father built their
home overlooking the Sacramento Valley, with a flagpole planted in
the front lawn that every passerby would be sure to see. Each morning
like clockwork, my grandfather raised the stars and stripes with pride,
and every evening they were retired until the next dawn.

The Army rejected my father for an abdominal injury when
he volunteered for the Vietnam War at age eighteen, and the Los

Angeles Police Department turned him down for the same reason at age nineteen. He became a successful carpenter and businessman within our community, but his dream to serve endured, and at age thirty-nine he was accepted into the Sacramento Sheriff's Training Academy, resulting in offers from the Los Angeles, Sacramento, and El Dorado County Sheriff's departments. My father and mother were involved in almost every step of my life, and with few exceptions, I relied on their counsel to guide my decisions and help me trust in my leaps of faith.

* * *

Katie and her family fly to New Orleans for my graduation. Her father's lung cancer has advanced, but despite the hardship, since we started dating, our families have grown closer. Our week is filled with celebration, food, and talk about our future. Everyone revels in the sights and sounds of the city, eating, toasting, and dancing the night away in the French Quarter. Katie and I are committed to our relationship, planning a life together in California. After I start my family medicine residency at Naval Hospital Camp Pendleton, she will move closer to me in San Diego and continue working in sports media advertising.

My graduation is held in a New Orleans theater downtown. After speeches conclude, we parade down the center aisle with Mardi Gras umbrellas held high, dancing to music and waving to the crowd like rock stars. I grin with excitement as my family and Katie clap me down the aisle like a celebrity. I'm overjoyed to put on that white coat and start practicing my craft. The ceremony concludes for all graduates except those entering the military. We are escorted from the theater stage to a separate room on the side. It's a small room with white folding chairs, a small podium at the front right, and a desk in the center with official orders for each new officer to sign. We seat ourselves in a single row, and a naval officer enters the room, prompting us to stand at attention and raise our right hands as the oath of office is read aloud:

I, [name], do solemnly swear that I will support and defend the Constitution of the United States against all enemies, foreign and domestic; that I will bear true faith and allegiance to the same; that I take this obligation freely, without any mental reservation or purpose of evasion; and that I will well and faithfully discharge the duties of the office on which I am about to enter. So help me God.

Each of us responds in unison, "Yes sir, I will." That's it, short and sweet yet solidifying our future in the military for a minimum of seven years. I am officially a Lieutenant in the United States Navy. My heart swells with pride and accomplishment, yet I'm feeling a little uneasy, keenly aware my future in the Navy is uncertain. The horrific events of September 11th, 2001 are still fresh in my mind and there are rumors in military circles about a possible U.S. invasion. The rumors are only speculation but enough to make me feel edgy and on alert, curious what my future holds as my Navy commitment commences.

The next twelve months are packed from August 2002 to July 2003 are packed. I move to an apartment in Oceanside, California, a military town outside the gates of Camp Pendleton, mostly populated by Marine Corps and Navy personnel and their families. Camp

Pendleton is the largest Marine Corps base on the west coast, boasting an aircraft station, amphibious assault group, infantry battalions, and artillery units. It is the Corps' largest expeditionary land-to-sea training facility, and the essence of Navy-Marine Corps prowess. Miramar and Coronado are thirty minutes south, home of Topgun and Navy Seal training sites. It's all there to train the best, most advanced operational fighting force in the world. Combine this with eleven miles of undeveloped beautiful California coastline and you can't help but feel patriotic when you arrive. Katie lives forty minutes away in Old Town, San Diego. We talk every day and see each other as much as possible. She supports my every move, sacrificing her opportunities as a sports journalist to stay near me.

Picturing my life with her is easy; her relentless pursuit of happiness and fun are contagious. I feel calm and forget the challenges of internship when we're together, and I'm quickly falling in love with her. When we have time off, we hike, mountain bike, and take short trips. Our favorite destination is a small village called Puerto Nuevo south of the San Diego-Mexico border. From my apartment, we can make it there in two and a half hours for fresh lobster, homemade tortilla soup, guacamole, and margaritas, all for under fifty dollars. Katie will never let me miss out on a good time and it keeps me sane during my internship year. After a few more months, we are engaged and planning our future. I feel my life is full and everything is moving in the right direction.

The Naval Hospital is ten miles inland on Camp Pendleton. Since the 1960s it has cared for active duty members, veterans, and their families. The first year of training is my internship, the most demanding of any three-year residency. Working hours are long, typically twelve to fourteen per day, with on-call duty every third night and expectations to move fast, learn quickly, and not fall behind. I rotate through all medical specialties required of a family physician: internal medicine, obstetrics, gynecology, minor surgery, dermatology, pediatrics, neurology, geriatrics, and more, all designed to hone my skills as a physician and prepare me to practice independently. After my first six months of internship, I travel to San Antonio, Texas for combat medic training. During the four weeks, I study combat trauma and learn modern techniques in field care under fire and tactical patient evacuations. It concludes with a two-day mock war, designed to emulate live combat trauma with everything from simulated gunfire and mortars to wounded marines with moulage blast wounds and helicopter medevacs.

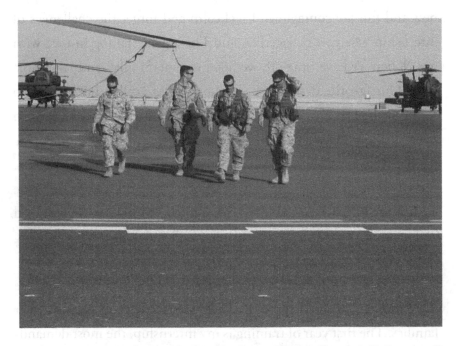

From left to right includes: Lt. Donnelly Wilkes, Lt. Cormac O'Connor, Corpsman #1, Corpsman #2

During the medical and field training, I often feel pushed to my limit, exhausted from the sheer number of hours on duty, and at the brink of my ability to retain information. Although I have transient doubts and worries about my ability to endure, the seeds never take root. My attitude remains positive, and I rebound quickly with renewed determination to bring on the next challenge. I have stars and stripes in my eyes, feeling that this life suits me. I like wearing my camouflage uniform, being in the field, and saluting the flag. I'm proud when I get to say, "I'm a naval officer and physician." I like the feeling of being pushed to the edge, even beyond my comfort zone, knowing I can recover and excel. At each phase of my training, I'm thinking about the future, optimistic but slightly uneasy about where I may end up. I feel like I've overcome serious obstacles to get to this point, but I'm craving more stability in my life. I know a military life doesn't fit this model, but I hope my time in the Navy will eventually be a means to this end.

In March of 2003, combined forces from the United States, the United Kingdom, Australia, and Poland invade Iraq. The main body encounters little resistance as the Iraqi Army is swiftly defeated and by April 9th, coalition forces occupy Baghdad. Saddam Hussein and central leadership go into hiding as U.S.-led occupying forces settle in. My internship year is nearing completion. We receive periodic updates on military operations at our monthly staff meetings. Tensions remain high especially in the Anbar Province to the west of Baghdad, but no orders have been passed down to mobilize or deploy.

My faith in God is strong and helps me to persevere, but it wasn't always that way. I was raised Roman Catholic, and my whole family has Catholic roots. I attended church and catechism regularly as a child and served as an altar boy. I liked it, but looking back, I realize I was mostly going through the motions. During high school, I knew something was missing, a disconnect with God on how my Catholic background fit into my life. I felt God's presence, but didn't know how to translate that into my world or connect it with others. I wondered constantly if I was doing good enough. I started to search, looking outside the Catholic Church, asking questions I had never asked about God. I started researching historical facts about Jesus and questioning Catholic rules and traditions. I knew I was supposed to love others, to follow God's word, but I worried what might happen if I made a terminal misstep, going beyond the point of no return to God's love. I read more books, firsthand stories about Jesus and facts about his life and teachings and found it was quite different from what I knew. My eyes and heart were opening, hearing the word of God in a new tone and seeing His presence with a softer lens. I wanted to know more.

After graduating high school, I worked at a drug store, where my new coworker invited me to a teen youth group at Green Valley Community Church. It was held on a Saturday night in the rec room at the church. The first night walking in, I was fascinated by the change of venue from the Catholic church. There was zero pressure, nobody cared where I came from or what I had done. I was simply welcomed. During group sessions, we talked about our lives and played games and sports in the gym. With a no-hassle approach, the youth leader helped break down walls and fears about Christianity, assuring me it's normal to have doubts, ask questions, and struggle in faith. In time, I learned that there is nothing I can do to lose God's love, nothing that is so egregious I can't find a way back, and I don't have to earn it, just accept it. What?! I was blown away. I felt God's presence in a new way, connecting with scripture in the Bible and literature from Christian scholars unlike before. I attended youth group regularly, and felt like a new chapter was opening for me, wearing my faith like a new pair of shoes that lightened my load. By the time I left for college at age twenty-one, I felt confident about my Christian faith and its place in my life; at the same time, I knew I was a rookie, still in the infancy of my faith. I expected to stumble and make mistakes and realized it requires work and growth to solidify a relationship with God, but I knew it was there for the taking if I wanted it.

Graduation from internship is scheduled for July 15th, 2003, confirming two milestones: I've passed my board examination and I am licensed to practice medicine as an independent physician. I'm feeling a sense of great accomplishment and confidence, but with this comes another fork in the road and yet another big decision. Following internship, I can choose one of three paths: First, continue residency at the hospital for two more years, finalizing all required training as a physician, then serve on active duty for four years. Second, leave residency to serve on active duty for two years with the Navy fleet (called going blue side), then return and complete residency. Third, leave residency to serve on active duty with the Marines for two years (called going green side), then return and complete residency.

Katie and I are weighing the pros and cons, including the war in Iraq, deployment cycles and locations, and attempting to stay near home. Ultimately, I make my choice, but it's only a "request" since it's up to the commanding officer to determine who goes where, and this is subject to the needs of the Navy. After much debate, I enter my request to go green side with the Marines, knowing this will give me the best chance to stay closest to Katie and allow her to remain at our townhome recently purchased in Oceanside. If granted, I'll be the battalion surgeon, one of two doctors assigned to care for roughly one thousand men in a battalion. I'll have fifty Navy corpsmen to help me provide primary medical care, both during training at Pendleton and during the deployment including combat missions. The infantry Marines are the tip of the spear; when it's go-time they will be called first, and if there is combat action, they will be there with Navy corpsmen alongside them. It's a decision I struggle with, knowing I may put myself in harm's way, but it's the best choice for my life and future with Katie.

Three weeks later new orders have been cut, and it's time to learn my assignment for the next two years. I'm called to the First Marine Division Headquarters at Camp Pendleton. I arrive early, wearing green digital camouflage, the same worn by Marine Corps personnel. I'm escorted into a small room with a desk at one end and three metal folding chairs in front, facing the desk. I'm asked to take a seat until Major Bradburn arrives. With nervous excitement, I sit in the cold metal chair with my naval service portfolio on my lap.

Major Bradburn walks into the room shortly, and I stand to attention saying, "Good afternoon, sir."

"Good afternoon, Lieutenant Wilkes," he replies quickly while taking his seat.

"I'll get right to the point, Lieutenant," he says. "Do you know why you're here today?"

"Yes sir, to receive new orders for my next duty station," I reply.

"Good, let's jump to it. You're going to be assigned to the Marine Corps infantry as the battalion surgeon, but we're still working out which medical officers will go where. We need two officers who are ready to potentially deploy in short order. I can't give you many details, but things are heating up in the Anbar Province outside of Baghdad, so this region may be your target."

"I understand, sir," I say, processing every word.

"I know you just graduated internship and there is a lot on your plate. I understand you've had excellent training and performed well in your rotations. I need to ask if you feel you're prepared to enter a battalion entering a rapid deployment cycle. Alternatively, we can consider assignment to a battalion that will remain stateside for at least a year."

Without explanation, his message is clear to me: we're going to war and his job is to find two doctors who are ready to deploy to a combat zone. He can't say this directly, but I understand the implications of the conversation. I only have seconds to draft a response in my head; it's something I did not expect to encounter today. I quickly reason that with the recent world events, I'll likely deploy soon no matter what; why not get it underway and get back home. It will be hard to bring this news home to Katie today, but I would rather get underway than sit idle.

After a moment, I reply, "Sir, I'm ready to go, I can handle it. Which battalion will I be assigned to?"

"Good to hear Lieutenant, you'll be joining First Battalion, Fifth Marines. We need two docs for this billet. Is there another medical officer from your class who you think would be a good fit?" he asks. "We need two guys who can gel together quickly and are prepared to go."

I don't hesitate with my reply. "Lieutenant O'Connor sir. I've known him for a long time, including medical school and internship. He's solid, and we get along very well. You'll have to ask him how he feels about it, but I recommend him."

"Excellent, I'll consider that. Thank you for your flexibility with this new assignment. You will be a strong asset to the battalion. Your new orders will be cut within twenty-four hours. Then you will be issued field gear and join the battalion at Camp Horno."

"Thank you, sir."

I stand and shake his hand. We depart the room in opposite directions.

As I open the double doors to walk down the steps of command headquarters, the mid-morning sun hits my eyes. I squint in the sunlight as my eyes adjust, pausing to look out at the grassy hills of Camp Pendleton. The smell of sagebrush permeates the air; Cobra helicopters echo in the distance—both have become familiar to me this past year. In this moment I feel my world has changed and the scenes around me take on a different feel; they now represent the place I'll be leaving and trying to come back to.

I'm feeling a rush of adrenaline like someone hit the turbo button and my body is the engine. I'm feeling excitement for a new adventure, yet edgy over the destination and rapid timeline. I need to talk to Katie, to tell her our future has changed and we need to make new plans.

We discussed many scenarios, but an early deployment was not one of them. I need to tell my family; my father will take the news seriously and proudly, understanding it must be done. However, I'm concerned my mother will be saddened and worried. She feels quite different about my decision to join the military, and she let my father know it. She believes my decision to join was an extension of his tendency to be an overbearing father with a bullish sense of duty.

It has been a source of contention since I started medical school and has been heightened since 9/11. I knew it worried her and caused them arguments. Regardless, I made my decision free and clear of their discord, understanding there would be hardships, but also much to gain: adventure, patriotism, and a way to pay for medical school.

As the implications of my new assignment run through my head, I'm wishing I could slow things down, take a step back, and reassess the situation. But I know my future has been set in motion, and new orders are coming down the pipe. I tell myself this is where I'm supposed to be, that I've done the best I can to control my destiny and the rest is out of my hands. That night, Katie and I share the news with laughter and tears. It's a twist we knew was possible, just not this soon. We are planning our wedding for the following year, but now it's indefinitely on hold. We spend the next few weeks strategizing our life apart, her job, and where she will live. We decide she will move into the townhome in Oceanside and continue working at *Transworld Skateboarding* magazine. After connecting with other military couples, we learn more about the challenges of deployment, namely uncertain timelines, difficulty with communication, and legalities like finances and wills. Internet and phone calls are limited, especially when deployed to a combat zone. Then one night I throw it on the table: "*Let's get married and not tell anyone.*" She looks at me with a smile and crinkle in her nose replying, "Yeah let's do it."

Within twenty-four hours, we enter the drive-through at A Little White Wedding Chapel in Las Vegas, Nevada. The menu includes an Elvis ceremony for an extra hundred dollars. I tell Katie to skip it and go for the budget package. After a few vows and signatures, we say "*I do,*" and just like that, on November 10th, 2003 we are married. We never tell anyone until right now in this book—surprise, family!

CHAPTER 2

Deploying to War, December 16, 2003

One month later it's past midnight when the doorbell rings at our townhome, just outside the gates of Camp Pendleton. D-Day has come for the Marines and Sailors of First Battalion, Fifth Marines. Historically, this is the day on which any important military operation is to begin. Now it commonly refers to June 6, 1944, during World War II, the day on which Allied forces invaded northern France using beach landings in Normandy. Today we commence our deployment to Okinawa, then Fallujah, Iraq. Katie and I had gone to bed early, hoping to sleep away the dread of our separation. Unsuccessful, we had been up for hours.

Opening the door, I see Lieutenant Cormac O'Connor and his wife Jen outside in the cold night air. They have forced friendly smiles on their faces and carry anticipation in their eyes. Our lives have paralleled each other for the last five years. Cormac is not only a fellow naval medical officer for this deployment but also a remarkably close friend. We both attended Tulane University School of Medicine and roomed together, completed internship training together, and now will go to war together. From the pool of deployment-ready physicians at Camp Pendleton, Cormac and I fit the bill.

We load my silver Toyota 4Runner and head for Camp Pendleton. The thirty-minute drive through the dark and deserted hills of Camp Pendleton is quiet and solemn. Since the days of World War II, men have trained and deployed for war on these grounds, and now it is my turn. I attempt to make small talk to take my mind off the fact I am leaving Katie for possibly up to ten months, but it is fruitless. As we drive, I feel a nervous ache in the pit in my stomach. I grip Katie's hand as we wind through the dark hills of Camp Pendleton to the home of First Battalion, Fifth Marines at Camp San Mateo. At 12:30 a.m., we pull up to the parade deck, a large asphalt parking lot where we will stage our gear, stand in formation, and say our goodbyes.

We drop our sea bags among a mountain of others and begin the waiting game. In the military, I had become grudgingly used to showing up extremely early for events, then waiting for unknown amounts of time for something to happen.

There is a chill in the air, turning wisps of breath into clouds as we talk huddled inside the 4Runner, waiting for the call to muster. The mood is somber, but we attempt to lighten it with sarcastic comments about life in the military and futures of fame and glory. I hold Katie's hand and do not let go as my thoughts drift.

The weeks leading to this day have been bittersweet. The holidays were filled with family and friends, home-cooked meals, and peaceful moments. It was wonderful; however, there were too many goodbyes, too many admonishments to "stay safe," and "watch your back." It amounted to an overwhelming urge to get the deployment underway. Katie and I felt blessed to have the unconditional support, but the emotional rollercoaster of leaving was draining and we felt the only resolution was to get the deployment underway.

Prior to our day of departure at Camp Pendleton, the battalion officers met in an old brick building with pale yellow walls, musty hallways, and a stale water fountain. A slide show with faded satellite pictures and mugshots of the top ten terrorists told me what to expect and to be prepared for the worst.

As battalion surgeons, Cormac and I are the primary care doctors for all the men, over nine hundred of them. As marines and sailors train for combat, we will provide all their primary care, treating illness, injury, and chronic medical conditions. Entering an infantry battalion as a medical officer requires training beyond that of traditional doctors, especially after only one year of internship. To understand the unique needs of military members and treat combat injuries, we are put through hours of field medical training and hands-on trauma scenarios, dramatized in live fashion. To accomplish this, throughout my four years of medical school, one year of internship, and months with the battalion, the Navy-Marine Corps alliance spares no expense. In Newport, Rhode Island, I spend six weeks learning the history of navy medicine, simulated ship duty, marching, and physical training, all designed to mold me into a naval officer. In San Antonio, Texas at the trauma lab, I practice intubations and control of massive hemorrhage on pigs, then camp for five days in the wilderness practicing field casualty care. At the Los Angeles County+USC Medical Center, I spend four weeks with the trauma team. During our twenty-four-hour shifts, gunshot wounds, stabbings, and car accident victims are all commonplace. I place chest tubes, surgical airways, and assist in open surgeries. At Camp Pendleton, we venture into the hills with Marine platoons in attack mode on nighttime raids. Gunfire, mortars, helos, and mock targets are all designed to emulate live combat scenarios and injuries. At each step, I'm elevating my skills, pushing myself to higher levels, and developing the confidence of an elite combat medic. I thrive in it, even hunger for it, knowing it's what I'll need to persevere in extreme situations, and save lives.

For deployment and combat operations, we are tasked to determine the medical supplies needed and coordinate field care, evacuations, and medical logistics for the entire battalion. We have fifty Navy corpsmen to help us. Some are assigned to platoons leaving the base on missions, others will remain at the medical aid station on base near Fallujah. If the battalion mobilizes from our base to attack Fallujah, we will pack our medical supplies to establish a field aid station near the front lines, receive injured marines, and treat combat wounds. Depending on the trajectory of the attack, we will adjust our location and distribution of corpsmen as needed.

The task is daunting, and as I sat through our dimly lit intelligence briefs, I imagined it had been the same for generations of military officers preparing for deployment in the profession of arms with well-meaning superiors putting forward their best efforts to ready their men for the inevitable.

I paid close attention to every word, every caution, and the lessons gained from those who had gone before me. I learned the essential equipment I must bring, and precautions I must take because wise military travelers before me told me so. I kept diligent notes that I referred to time and time again. Yet, beyond this, I sensed my predicament was an unknown, and as we planned, I became keenly aware that nothing could fully prepare me for embarking on the greatest undertaking of my life, an adventure of magnificent proportions, the kind where fantastic stories and heroes are born. What fortunes awaited me only God surely knew. As I continued to plan and prepare for deployment, my imagination ran wild.

I'm jolted back to the task at hand. From across the street, a marine with a bullhorn voice yells for all personnel to muster into formation and load the buses. Cormac and I reluctantly step out of the 4Runner, pair off with our wives, and say our final goodbyes. I'm gripped by sadness and struggle to look into her eyes knowing I will not see her for up to ten months. As I hold her close, the dark hills surround me and the cold night grips me as my sadness deepens. We both make promises to call and write when we can, but I feel her tears against my face.

When I sense I can stay no longer, I give her a final kiss goodbye, let go of her hand, and walk away. Cormac and I join the ranks of our men and then, in single file, board the whitewashed school buses. We take our seats and tuck our day packs between our legs. Each man counts off out loud, and when the last man has sounded off, the platoon commander gives the "all present and accounted for" signal. The diesel-powered buses roar to life and lurch forward, taking us away from our base, and me away from the girl I love. I press my forehead to the foggy window to look for her, but she is already gone.

Our destination is a two-hour drive to March Air Reserve Base in Riverside County, California. Eighty miles up the road is Barstow, California. Barstow is one of those high desert towns you only pass through on the way to somewhere else—the kind with crappy coffee and good people-watching at the gas station. When I was young, our family used to pass through Barstow on the way to Lake Mojave for our annual family waterskiing trip. We usually stopped at McDonald's for a bathroom break and lunch. It had an old train car they'd made into a dining area and I always thought it would be neat to eat our lunch in that train car. But usually we were too rushed to stop and sit for our meal, so we just ate in the car. As we rumble toward March and Barstow in the big whitewashed buses, it occurs to me once again that I will not be stopping, nor having my lunch in that train car because again I'm on my way to somewhere else.

At March, we exit the buses and file into a large hanger. It is a reception area for returning or outgoing marines and sailors. It is filled with tables piled with muffins and magazines; packaged sandwiches that look too old to eat; and refrigerators with water, orange soda, or red juice drinks. There are rows of folding chairs set up for us to rest and large silver dispensers filled with hot coffee. There is fanfare with streamers and "welcome home" banners proclaiming a job well done. I long to be the returning party instead of the one heading outbound, and I cannot help but feel jealous of the returning members who have already served their time.

After a failed attempt to stay awake, I find a spot among the marines to lie facedown on the cement floor with my pack beneath my head as a pillow. I pass out for what seems like mere seconds, only to be woken by a sergeant yelling, "Okay, everyone up and into formation; let's move!"

Clumsily, I gather my belongings and file out to the jetway, where I'm amazed to see our marines and sailors climbing into a large Continental Airlines plane. We lumber up the stairway with our packs and weapons and, to my surprise, I find myself seated in first class with a television and a fully reclining chair. Since joining the Marines, I have never done or seen anything remotely approaching the pampering of "first class." The marines generally pride themselves on doing more with less. Our high-class accommodations are a welcome extravagance I gladly accept for the long flight from southern California to Okinawa, Japan, the first stop on my journey.

As weariness takes hold of me during the flight, questions enter my mind. "Will I survive the trials that lie ahead?" "Am I strong and brave enough?" I want to drift off to sleep, but I am pessimistic, and unknowns cloud my confidence. The skeptic inside me questions what I will gain from this deployment but hardship. Will it make me a better man? I selfishly feel I have already endured my share of trials, and then there is Katie—I can't think about her without terrible sadness.

There are no present answers to my questions. As I sit in my chair, my head resting in my hands, looking out at the limitless darkness, I realize I have up to twelve months of deployment ahead of me and time is my enemy. I listen to the jet engines moaning in synchronicity. We fly through the night, jetting towards unknown and violent parts of the world; home may as well be ten thousand miles away. Then the plane turns, and a thrust of power pushes the nose upward, rousing my confidence once more. As the plane climbs, my spirits begin to lift. Perhaps this experience will refine me as a doctor, fulfill my sense of duty, and quench my thirst for adventure as my move to New Orleans did. Still, I question my path at this point in my life. The timing seems horrible. Katie and I are now secretly married and there is no firm date of return. Katie's father recently passed away after fighting lung cancer, and his absence left a hole in the family that can never be filled. He meant the world to Katie, and I lament that in a short time, I am the second man to leave her unexpectedly.

My heart is heavy and I'm feeling torn, wrestling with the choices that have put me in desert boots and on a plane to the Middle East. This was nowhere in the Navy brochure when I signed up before entering medical school; the recruiters don't mention combat. I reason it is my heartfelt service to God and country that has led me to this crossroads, and for better or for worse it is what I have been chosen to do. I'm ready to jump in the ring and give my service. I'm trying hard to put my faith in God, believing He will protect me. I reason I will give Him my time in exchange for His protection and guidance. I know it's flawed and just doesn't work that way, but right now, sitting on a plane at thirty thousand feet, it's the best I can do.

PRIVATE ERIKSON & OKINAWA

The first destination for 1st Battalion, 5th Marines (1/5) is Okinawa, Japan. Our purpose on Okinawa is to refine urban combat training in preparation for the fight we will face in Iraq. Small Iraqi villages have been constructed to simulate live combat scenarios. Lectures, intel briefs, and live-fire drills consume the days. We are stationed at Camp Hansen, one of seven Marine Corps camps on Okinawa. Its establishment in the aftermath of World War II allowed the United States to maintain sovereignty over the island and other parts of Japan.

I spend my days at the medical clinic, caring for Marines injured during training exercises and performing many administrative duties. In the evenings, I watch DVDs at the barrack, go to the base gym, and mingle with the Marine Corps officers. Although we come from different worlds, infantryman versus medicine man, our mission in Iraq is the same, and as the weeks pass, bonds form. We share in the hardships of training for war, and in short order these men I have only known for a few months are my close friends.

The island training is intense, and there is little night life for the Marines. We all know where we are heading, and at times the boredom leads to problems. As I sit in my office at the Battalion Aid Station on an afternoon nearing our day of departure to Iraq, I get a knock on my door.

"Enter!" I say loudly to rise above the clamor of corpsmen working outside in the clinic.

The door pushes open and a Marine walks in. He is dressed in desert cammie uniform and his head is turned down to the floor. He closes the door behind him, stands directly in front of me, and lifts his eyes to meet mine. His name is Private Erikson.

"Sir, can I talk to you?" He says calmly but with an air of concern.

"Sure you can. My door is always open, private," I reply.

"My platoon commander told me I have to talk with you," he says, then pauses as if he is going to speak again but stops short.

I give him a chance to start again, but when he hesitates, I say, "Well, I'm sure he sent you here for a reason, so I'm all ears."

This isn't the first time we have met; we know each other from Pendleton. Physically, he is a poster boy Marine. He stands nearly six feet tall and walks with a long, smooth strut. He is solid from head to toe, and his shoulders are stacked like blocks. The most striking feature is his brick house jaw that frames his face. His eyes are calm and blue and he carries himself with confidence, yet he is the type of guy who always lives on the edge.

The first time I met Private Erikson, we were at Camp Pendleton at the battalion medical clinic. I had seen him a few times for a knee injury he was nursing back to health. I counseled him on some stretching and strengthening exercises, and he followed up with me in clinic as instructed. He was always polite and well groomed, and he seemed to have the respect of his fellow Marines; at the same time, I could tell he was different from other marines. He had an air of respectful confidence when speaking to me and was not intimidated when talking to officers.

He spoke rather freely and cracked jokes. I could tell he was the center of attention among his fellow marines, a rebel in his mind, and I suspect he liked it that way.

Today, however, his demeanor is off. He didn't walk in with the same tone and posture, so I can tell something is wrong. He isn't sure how to start the conversation, so I ask him, "Private, how is the training going? Are you ready to get the heck out of here like I am?"

"Hell yes, sir." He quickly replies as his eyes perk up.

"I know this training is important for you guys, but the boredom is killing us all," I say.

"That's for damn sure, sir," he confidently announces. "The thing is, that's why my platoon commander sent me to see you. I did something pretty stupid, and I'm worried I could get kicked out of my platoon."

"Okay, tell me what happened," I encourage him.

"I can't lie, sir, these past few weeks, the long hours have been getting to me, especially at night. There's only so much time I can spend at the gym, at the chow hall, or playing video games. After a while, I just go stupid crazy with boredom," he explains.

"I understand, private, and I guarantee you're not alone. We're all ready to get off this island, and as crazy as it sounds, I want to go to Iraq more than I ever thought possible. I want to get this mission over with just like you, but that doesn't explain why your platoon commander sent you here," I press.

He pauses for a moment, his eyes peer around at the painted block walls and old linoleum floor typical of many Marine Corps buildings, and then he calmly begins to unbutton the cuff of his left cammie-sleeve. I have no idea what he is going to show me until I see the bandages covering his forearms as he rolls up his sleeves. He stands with his arms extended towards me and sighs with a look of frustration on his face as he says, "Well, sir, you see, last night the intensity of my boredom was just too much and I took my Ka-Bar and sliced my arms up. I know it was stupid, and I only did it for the hell of it. It's just that…we can't do anything here—we can't go out, we can't drink, I'm bored off my ass."

As I process what he is telling me, I keep the conversation going. "Private, you know how concerning this looks, right? The command takes this type of thing very seriously. Tell me what else is going on. How are you getting along with your platoon; how are you sleeping and eating; how are your spirits?"

"All that is fine, sir," he replies without hesitation. "This was just an off night that had been building, and I needed something to…you know, to help me feel alive."

"I get that, private, but this doesn't look like just boredom. We need you to be one hundred percent once we enter the combat zone. Fellow marines are depending on you. We have many hard months to go, and this island is just the beginning, so if something is weighing you down, now is the time to tell me. This is a safe place to do it, and it won't affect your deployment as long as we get it on the table and address it now."

He does not reply right away and takes a moment to sit down in the chair behind him. He cuffs his hands in his lap, looks up at me, and says, "Sir, I know I can be impulsive at times and this looks bad. But I am good to go, and this will never happen again. I need to stay with my unit."

I believe him. During my examination, he does not show any signs of depression or harmful or suicidal thoughts. I stand up and walk to him. He stands up as well. I calmly say, "I think you're an excellent marine, one of the best in your unit. I know this deployment is going to bring some challenges that will make your head spin. Rely on your training, your instinct, and your fellow men when the going gets tough. This incident is no different; learn from it and make yourself stronger. I don't think it will happen again, but if you run into trouble, come talk to me, agree?"

A smile of relief comes across his face. "Yes, sir, I will," he calmly replies.

"Now, you understand I have to get you cleared by Psych, but I'll make darn sure he knows who you are," I tell him.

"Got it, sir. thank you," he replies.

"You bet, I'll see you in Iraq, private." He smiles, nods, and exits the door. I lean back in my creaky desk chair, watching him walk away. I believe he knows everything will be okay, that I will take care of him, and he can endure. "Good Lord," I think, "we haven't even landed in Iraq yet and already the pressures are pushing guys to the brink."

Oddly enough, he was insightful about the stupidity of his actions and regretted all the trouble he had caused. There were no further incidents, and when I spoke with his company commander about the situation, he told me Private Erikson was one of the most outstanding marines he's ever worked with. Over the next few months, before Private Erikson and I would conclude our deployment and part ways for good, we would meet again at two climactic events, both defining moments in our lives.

The final days of training in Okinawa wind down, and after two and a half months, we finally leave for Iraq. Our destination is

Fallujah, in the Anbar Province. The Marines' mission is to fall in and take over all military operations in Fallujah and the surrounding territory, an area currently controlled by U.S. Army personnel. The region has recently become unstable, and the Marines have been ordered to take command and restore order. My mission is to coordinate and provide first-level medical care for all the marines and sailors in our battalion, nearly one-thousand men. Our forward operating base (FOB) is positioned a few miles from the outer limits of Fallujah, and, at this stage in the war, it is the most violent place in Iraq.

CHAPTER 3

The Convoy, March 18th, 2004 (Day of Departure + 93)

I awake at 1:30 a.m. in the back of our Humvee ambulance, just after we cross the border into Iraq. This is the first leg of our three-day convoy from the safety of Kuwait into the unknowns of Iraq. Sleep has been erratic, punctuated by bumps in the road, jolts off the highway, and moaning metal. The back of the ambulance is cold, green, and sterile. It holds four stretchers, two on the bottom and two suspended from above. You can walk down the center aisle for access to each patient. My rucksack hangs next to me, and in it I brought essentials: toothbrush, towel, shave kit, change of clothes, a book about the Middle East, and some packaged snacks. Nylon straps, intravenous fluid bags, and clear plastic tubing hang from the ceiling, gently swaying over my head as the top-heavy truck grumbles down the highway. The smell is musty, typical of military vehicles, lending an odd but familiar comfort.

I am wide awake, with thoughts stirring and a curious dark world outside. It's cold as I poke my head out of my Navy-issued forest green sleeping bag. All I hear is a mixed chorus of winding from our engine, big knobby tires thundering over asphalt and the creaking metal walls of the ambulance carriage. It is black except for the flicker of headlights coming through the windshield of the main cabin. I sit up on the stretcher, swinging my legs onto the floor. I hang a red flashlight from the ceiling; dust particles flicker as they catch the light and drift towards the floor. I pull out some sanitary wipes and clean the grime from my arms and face, then put them in a pile next to me. My eyes shift to the ground, and I see a small beetle scurry across the floor. I pull on my desert brown boots and grab an extra jacket from my pack, then a green apple and a hard granola bar. Leaning into the forward cabin, I peer out the window and see the taillights of each vehicle ahead of us. Otherwise, there is only limitless darkness. Our convoy is spaced fifty yards per truck, heading northbound on one of the main artery highways towards Baghdad. Snaking along in the night, stopping at various checkpoints for gas, food, and supplies, we move deeper into the heart of an ancient land. The bulk of travel is on unimproved asphalt highways, with unpredictable stretches of gravel, crumbled cement, and caked dirt flats. Like a world after nuclear fallout, the land is barren, cracked, and devoid of life.

Two of my corpsmen sit up front, one driving, the other navigating and keeping coms with the convoy commander. As I shuffle closer to the portal connecting the patient bay to the main cabin, I hear them talking softly. Their voices are a welcome comfort, and I poke my head up into the cabin to ask how they are doing. Petty Officer Williams holds a map of the region in his lap and points out our location with a small handheld flashlight. We are about one hundred miles across the border, and as I look ahead, I see the lights of our convoy stretching for miles, surrounded by infinite darkness. I gaze off to the west and on the horizon I see flickers of light. As we come closer, the lights are brighter, and I realize these flickers are the flames of oil rigs blazing out of control. Huge clouds of billowing black smoke pour from each one, adding an even more sinister beauty to the night. These towering flames are the images I had seen on CNN when Saddam intentionally lit his oil rigs on fire. I am struck now that when I saw those television pictures from the comforts of my own home, never would I have dreamt that I would be driving towards them.

We travel north from Kuwait for three days across that ashen scabland, stopping only for gas and sleep. Signs of life are rare, no rivers or streams in sight, only miles of lifeless tortured earth. The ground is dry and broken, the slightest breath of wind whisks dirt into the air.

Small dilapidated towns punctuate the land. Humans wander in the background, peeking their heads from doors and windows as we pass. Amid the emptiness mingles the occasional goat herder, a field of withered crops, or a piecemeal clay hut. As we pass through, I'm struck at how lonely it feels, like an old west ghost town.

On the third day, we enter Anbar Province, the location of our forward operating base, Camp Mercury. With a population of over 1.5 million, and sharing borders with Syria, Jordan, and Saudi Arabia, it is the largest of Iraqi provinces. The convoy is successful, with only a few interruptions for IEDs (improvised explosive devices), but no enemy contact. I am exhausted and grateful to reach our base, where I have a roof over my head and warm food waiting. This is our home for the next four months. We are located a few miles from Fallujah, about an hour from Baghdad. The camp is one half mile in circumference with four unequal sides, previously one of Saddam's terrorist training camps before U.S. forces took it over. The perimeter is a poorly constructed stone wall in a rectangular shape, with a guard tower at each corner of the camp. Within the walls are a few simple hardened buildings built when it was inhabited by the Iraqis. These are now used as workspaces, while others beyond repair are used for storage. The remaining structures are tents left standing by the Army, now being replaced by the Marines since the region has become unstable. The tents are used for sleeping quarters, communications equipment, internet, and a small gym with weights. The ground is a mixture of fine ash-like dirt and gravel.

The Marines store water in large tanks that supply a shower trailer that accommodates about eight men. When the water in the tanks runs out, we either shower outdoors in open wooden structures or use bottled water to rinse in the shower trailer. The base operation staff place pallets of bottled drinking water at strategic areas around camp to help discourage dehydration. The water is boiling hot in the heat of the day but cools nicely in the evening.

Marine toilets are standard plastic outhouses. When you do your business, you better do it in the morning or evening; otherwise, you suffer the consequence of sitting in an outhouse that has cooked in the relentless blazing sun.

The chow hall is an old building that doubles as a chapel. A group of Marines truck in the hot food each day. They travel five miles to a larger base, pick up the food in large vats, and bring it back to our base for serving; this is carried out three times daily, feeding hundreds of men.

The food is decent considering where we are, but like anything done with forced repetition, the meals lose their appeal after a while. When hot food isn't available, we eat MREs (meals ready to eat). These prepackaged military meals are issued during combat operations or training exercises when Marines are living in the field and don't have access to hot chow. MREs are high in calories and salt and limited in flavor, but overall, most of the men agree they are a hearty and welcome meal when there isn't any other option.

Our Battalion Aid Station (BAS) is located inside one of the larger, older buildings. We stock basic medical supplies to take care of routine sick call needs, minor injuries, and some advanced equipment to stabilize more extensive trauma victims. We also construct a small room with plywood and wood studs to house our pharmacy supplies. Each corpsman is allotted a specified amount of medications, including morphine, valium, and anti-chemical warfare injection syringes to take on missions. Before deployment, the entire battalion is vaccinated against anthrax and smallpox, since there are still rumors of chemical warfare. For accessibility purposes, Cormac and I work and sleep in a small back room attached directly to the BAS. This is our new base and new home, and within a matter of hours, we are unloaded, unpacked, and ready for business.

CHAPTER 4

And So It Begins, March 23rd, 2004 (+ 98)

The first three days at Camp Mercury are uneventful, and I am beginning to settle into a routine at my new home. However, in short order, the true reality of our situation becomes known. It is the evening of March 23rd, 2004. After finishing my dinner, I head to the recreation tent to play ping-pong. Captain Jamie McCall, Captain Mike Butler, and I had been talking up our ping-pong skills since arriving at Camp Mercury, heatedly debating who is the best player. The rec tent is at the back of the camp, housing a ping-pong table, four televisions, board games, and books. I challenge Jamie in the first game and take a disappointing first round loss but come back strong in the second. As we play, marines come and go, some stop to talk and check out the commotion. We all wear Marine Corps green nylon shorts with cotton t-shirts and carry our weapons as mandated by the commanding officer. The sound of video games buzzes in the back of the tent where Marines enjoy the latest Xbox or Nintendo technology. On the other side of the tent is a forty-inch television surrounded by young

Marines watching *Animal House*, a classic comedy with the late John Belushi that I realize I have never seen.

As I sit next to the ping pong table watching Jamie and Mike go back and forth, I hear a distant rumble outside, like a thundercloud declaring its intentions before the storm. The rumbling ceases and I say nothing, but my curiosity perks up because it is a new sound, one I didn't recognize. I turn my head left to look at Cormac sitting next to me, and then, kaka-BOOM! As if a lightning bolt struck the tent, the concussive force throws us off balance onto the floor. Mass commotion ensues as we scramble to our feet and run towards the exit.

We scramble out the door and run for a hardened structure or building, just as we had been trained to do. I grab onto Cormac's sleeve, stumbling as I run behind him. In the chaos, I left my pistol, cammie blouse, and radio in the tent. I quickly decide they aren't worth going back for. As we clamor across the loose gravel in darkness, I feel one mortar after another pummeling the ground just beyond the walls of our base. Men scurry in all directions as the blast waves rattle my brain.

I yell to Cormac, "Damn it, let's get to the nearest building!"

He replies, "No, we have to get to the Battalion Aid Station!"

I don't have time to argue and the aid station is close, so I hold on tight and we make our way through the gravel, confusion, and darkness to the BAS, bursting through the doors. My heart pounds and head spins as I lean forward panting, taking inventory of what just happened.

As we storm into the BAS I yell to the corpsmen, "Get on your Kevlar and flak jacket and get the ambulance team ready to go!" I'm not sure if any mortars landed inside the compound, but we need to be ready if there are any casualties. The incoming mortars stop, but I can hear outbound counter artillery at Camp Fallujah just two miles away. They can track the trajectory of incoming fire and respond with outgoing rounds in the same direction.

In the BAS we gear up with medical supplies while our medical chief obtains accounts for all our men. I hustle to my room and stuff my medical pack with extra gauze, pressure bandages, splints, and morphine. My corpsmen are doing the same, unsure of how many marines may be wounded. My heart pounds in my chest as I try to keep a clear head. Everyone is accounted for; we gather around the radio to receive word of casualties. The walkie-talkie squawks to life as we move in closer.

"Attention all personnel, at this time no mortars have landed in the compound, and no injuries are reported. Maintain your posts for further orders."

I look to my left and then to my right; I take a step back and exhale a sigh of relief. We just survived our first attack.

This is our fourth day on the base. Intelligence informs us these mortars landed closer to the outer walls than ever before. Two days prior, seven medical personnel were wounded, and a doctor was killed from mortar attacks only two miles away at Camp Fallujah. I knew we would see action in Fallujah, but we just arrived! Fortunately, the insurgent mortar attacks lack precision; the mortars are fired from outdated or even homemade launchers, often from the backs of pickup trucks with a point and shoot strategy. Without radar or night vision technology, they frequently miss their targets. But when landed within five hundred yards, the ferocity of this weapon is not lost, and the explosion is terrifying, like nothing I've ever felt.

Despite my training and preparations, this is all so foreign to me, and I feel defenseless because I can't fight back. I'm pissed but there's nothing I can do about it, so I sit on the floor with the other corpsmen and quietly say prayers.

I pray for strength and resilience, for the courage to remain strong to lead my men. My efforts are honest and true, but I'm suffocating in doubt, feeling the vulnerability of what just happened. Cormac brings out some cards and suggests we play gin rummy. I numbly stare at my cards, moving them in my hands, half-heartedly going through the motions. I play one game, but I'm feeling restless and too agitated to continue, I lean forward and place my head in my hands.

The fact that we've been attacked is not a surprise; we expected it sooner or later, but no one can tell you "Hey, be prepared on the fourth night to get knocked off your ass by mortars." All the training in the world can't prepare you for that moment. I stand up and step out of the room to gather my composure. Rage runs through my mind. Right or wrong, I want their destruction—I want to be on the attack. From our intel briefs, I learned our enemy has many faces, some are insurgents also known as former regime elements, essentially Saddam loyalists continuing to fight in the name of Islam and Saddam. Others are Al Qaeda terrorists and mercenaries from countries like Syria and Iran who are paid to carry out hit-and-run style attacks, like the one we just endured. Finally, there are common thieves and criminals paid by insurgents to carry out specific missions. I know they want me dead at any cost, and the mortar attacks have brought this to life. These thoughts run through my mind like a pack of wild dogs. For the first time in my life, I feel what it's like to have someone try to kill me, and I want to kill them too. It is terrifying. I'm scared, and I hate knowing they have this power over me.

As I lie in my bed that night, emotions bombard me. I think a lot about my family, and I think about Katie. How will I explain this to them? What will I say? In one instant, I desperately want to talk to them and tell them what I've seen and heard. But in the next moment, I doubt if I can ever describe my new feelings of loneliness, hatred, and fear. After all, I think, what good will it do? It will only burden them with worry, and so I decide to record my thoughts in my journal and keep faith with God and my fellow men.

Later I drift off to sleep after exhausting myself with thoughts of the day's events. At 2:30 a.m., my eyes pop open from the sound of another blast. I lie stiff in my rack, staring straight up into the dark. At first, I think it might have been a dream. Cormac speaks up. "Donnelly, was that was another attack?…It sounded close."

Frustrated, I say, "I think so…I wonder if these bastards are going to keep this up all night. Why can't we stop them?" I know it's a question without an answer; there is nothing we can do, and no more words are said.

I take down my flak jacket from the shelf, open it up, and place it at the head of my bed, like a square with only three walls so my head lies at the entrance. This is my protection for the rest of the night in case a blast comes through the ceiling—an unlikely event, but anything seemed possible at this point. Eventually, I drift off to sleep again with my head against the metal plates of my flak jacket.

The rest of the night is quiet, but it's not long until they strike again. They hit us the next night with rockets that impact within five hundred yards of our compound. The rocket blast is so powerful, it feels like it lands right outside the BAS where I sleep.

While I knew other camps are getting mortared, I didn't expect the attacks to begin so soon after our arrival. I ask Captain Mike Butler about the frequency of the attacks since we arrived. He explains that some of it is luck, but a large part of it is very planned. The insurgents can see a large convoy rolling into town; they know we are turning over control of the region with the Army and that our counter measures and offensive operations will decrease from the normal cycle. They take advantage of this short intermission. He assures me that our boys will be locked on soon enough, patrolling the area and taking the fight to them.

Over the next few days, our battalion continues to settle in and take over military operations within the area. For each section of our battalion, this involves three phases. The first three to five days are spent meeting our counterparts, discussing their experiences and lessons learned during their deployment and observing how they operate daily. The next week, each member takes a more active role in his job, working side by side with his counterpart in a right seat, left seat fashion to ensure a seamless transition of operations.

For the medical section, we start work in the Battalion Aid Station, sending out daily medical situation reports and taking care of new patients. The marines take over battle positions, ride together on convoys, and go out on foot patrols. The final phase involves the official transfer of authority to our battalion and assumption of all duties. The departing members remain present in the background for a few days to assist. It isn't perfect but it gives each member the best chance of success while assuming an enormous amount of responsibility in an unknown and hostile environment over a short amount of time. As those of us living on camp get used to our new lives many other marines and sailors settle into ever more dangerous positions in the surrounding cities like Ramadi and Al-Garma.

For those of us on our first tour in Iraq, these first few days are an onslaught of trials and emotions, each one of us taking it in strides, consuming it, and adapting as best we can. As a unit, we are tackling the mission with immense coordination of effort and support for one another; as individuals, the processing is much more personal, and I'm feeling the weight of this burden.

CHAPTER 5

Emotions Take Hold, April 2nd, 2004 (+108)

As the days pass and life unfolds in my desert home, I accept the fact it is not a matter of if our boys will be injured but when. This timing takes care of itself within the first week. After chow on the morning of March 28th, 2004, the battle captain pulls me aside to tell me a Marine is en route back to our base with a shrapnel wound to his upper body. These are the only details he has about his condition. Apparently, one of our vehicles among a convoy heading through Al-Garma came under attack with grenades and small arms fire. One of the grenades landed ten feet behind this marine's Humvee and threw shrapnel in the back of it where he stood. I head towards the BAS to await his arrival and my stomach churns with anxious anticipation as this will be the first wounded marine of our deployment.

The convoy rolls in about 8:30 p.m. with our wounded man. As soon as they come through the BAS doors, there is a gaggle of people trying to get a look, and I tell my chief to take on crowd control. They bring him into the clinic and lay him on a stretcher. He looks about eighteen or nineteen years old. He has brownish-blond hair matted to his forehead with sweat and hazel-blue eyes that stand out on his face smeared with dirt and grease. His cammies are ripped open down his left forearm where I find some bloody gauze wrapped with tape. He is surrounded by a group of concerned marines and a familiar scent of dirt, gasoline, and sweat emanating from the group. As we move him off the stretcher, he winces with pain but seems in good condition despite his wounds.

I quiz him about his injuries while the corpsmen go to work cleaning the blood off his skin. He reports moderate pain from his shrapnel wounds, dizziness, and a pounding headache. I perform a thorough neurological exam and determine he does not have any deficits to warrant a CAT scan. His shrapnel wounds are mostly minor, with only a few small breaks in the skin and one larger puncture wound of his left forearm that requires more attention. After irrigating and exploring this wound with forceps, I realize it is deeper than I suspected and extends into the muscle compartment of his forearm. Cormac and I work on him together, irrigating it, then sewing multiple layers of sutures deep to superficial, with a tube-like drain left protruding from the skin. This is a small rubber tube set deeper into the wound space to drain fluids and help avoid infection. We keep the sutures loose and leave the top layer of the skin open to heal from the inside out. This will leave a larger scar but decrease the chance of infection of this dirty wound.

I watch his face as we work on him. He is quiet and unresponsive to the intermittent shouts of praise from his fellow marines in the background; he stares straight ahead with a glazed look over his face. I suspect his injuries have been quite a shock. He asks if he can call his wife, so we bring him a satellite cell phone. I can only imagine how difficult it will be to explain to his wife he's been wounded on one of his first missions, then expect to hang up and go on like any other day. The battalion commander stops by and tells him he will be back out with his men as soon as possible. He is given a ten-day course of antibiotics, and we remove the drain from his forearm two days later. I instruct his company corpsmen to watch him closely for signs of infection and have him perform daily physical therapy exercises to avoid loss of function of his hand muscles. He recovers well and returns to full duty within two weeks. He is our first wounded marine.

*   *   *

It's minutes before dawn when it happens; 5:20 a.m. as I'm sleeping deeply, my guard down for only moments when *WHAM!* A head-shaking thunderclap breaks my sleep, shattering all I know of rest and peace. I rise sharply in my bed, on the defense, frightened and cussing. My body stiffens and my head twitches in all directions. I cuss them for having the power to terrorize me, and I cuss them because I can't do anything about it. The mortar attacks have been increasingly frequent the last few days, which only makes them harder to bear.

I'm getting used to the interruptions of my life; however, the intensity of my emotions has been getting the best of me lately, a problem I had not anticipated. I have been quick tempered, irritable, and short with my corpsmen. I've felt a seething hatred for the enemy I had not known before. "Those F-ing bastards!" is what I've been calling them after the last few attacks. This hatred is simmering below the surface and starting to affect me in ways I'm unsure how to handle. I need an outlet, but what and how is unknown to me. My only solution is to grin and bear it until I figure out another way to deal with it.

I decide I want to know more about the people we are fighting. In my spare time, I read about the history of this ancient land, all the way back from biblical roots to the recent centuries of war and unrest. The insurgents are crafty; I can't see them or hear them until they land hell on our doorstep, firing rockets and mortars from seemingly nowhere. At our weekly intelligence meetings, I learn they are building make-shift rocket and mortar launchers from lead pipes, mounted and fired in the back of ordinary pickup trucks. The insurgents drive in at night on remote dirt roads, bringing themselves within attack range of our base. They fire off their munitions and scurry away. Their mortars can be fired from up to two thousand meters away, while the rockets have a range of five to ten miles. It's exceedingly difficult to defend against these attacks, and the U.S. military has been adjusting tactics as we learn. There is an immense span of ground that has to either be constantly patrolled or decorated with ambushes to catch them in the act. Our enemy is watching and learning our patterns, playing cat and mouse, and using time to their advantage. It takes a tremendous amount of energy, resources, and risk from our marines to maintain the patrols and presence to stop or catch them. I have great confidence in our leaders and their resolve to beat this enemy, but despite this, I'm realizing there is only so much we can do. I was naïve to this until to now. Despite all my training being in the military for nearly two years, I'm thinking "What the hell, we're the United States military, you can't get away with this." Now the truth is becoming clear.

This is war and anything goes. You can't predict or control it; the enemy will always find new ways to hurt you no matter how advanced your forces are. This is their home turf, and it's always been that way.

Our base is positioned a few miles from Fallujah, a city of approximately 250,000 residents located thirty-six miles west of Baghdad.

Fallujah has become the most volatile region in Iraq since early April 2003, and as a result has experienced violent crowd control incidents, murders, and bombings. The emergence of Fallujah as a seat of Sunni resistance is explained by the fact that many of its inhabitants are followers of the Wahhabi sect, a traditional Sunni extremist tribal clan that has occupied Fallujah for quite some time, going back into the 1990s, perhaps even into the 1980s. Of the 250,000 inhabitants, it is estimated that the insurgency totals around 20,000. Since our arrival at Camp Mercury, rumors have been circulating that something big is going down in Fallujah sooner than expected. It's becoming very apparent our battalion was sent to Fallujah for a strategic reason, and little time will be wasted getting down to the business of stabilizing this region. At our operations briefs, I've received intel of a strategic position near Fallujah called "the cloverleaf", and that it will be an emanant part of my future.

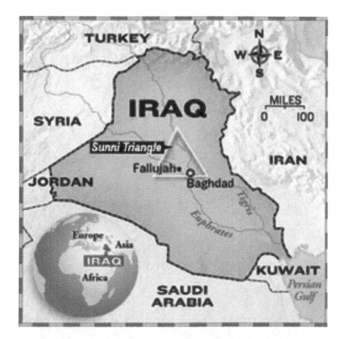

CHAPTER 6

Offensive Actions, April 4th, 2004 (+ 110)

Before the offensive in Fallujah begins, the staff officers are called together for a meeting with the Commanding General of 1st Marine Division, General James Mattis. Mattis led the 1st Marine Division during the early stages of the Iraq War, establishing himself as a premier field commander. He is known for his intellectualism as a career Marine, and as a straight shooter and a hard hitter in combat. He is here to outline the role our battalion will play in the assault and to show his support prior to engaging the enemy. Cormac and I attend the meeting at the Command Operations Center (COC) at our base two days before the attack is set to begin. The COC is in a tattered cinderblock building at the center of our base. We gather in a medium-sized room with a long table running down the center, folding chairs on all sides, and lots of maps on the yellow block walls. A projector is mounted overhead that illuminates the battlefield of Fallujah on the wall in front of us. A coffee maker perks in the corner next to a table loaded with snacks and drinks. I sit against the wall and wait with nervy excitement for the meeting to begin. Usually, there is more small talk and gesturing among the officers before the start of these weekly meetings, but this one is more serious. Insurgents have dug into Fallujah, and now the Marines are going in head-on with the intent of retaking the city and killing anyone who opposes them. Since the Marines are moving into battle, this means our medical support will need to move with them, and I am antsy to see the blueprint for where we will be positioned.

The meeting commences in typical Marine fashion: a door opens in the back of the room and someone yells, "Attention on deck!" Everyone springs up, standing at attention as General Mattis walks into the room. He tells us to take our seats as he proceeds to one end of the table. He is about five feet, nine inches tall with shortly trimmed, predominantly grey hair. His face has a fair complexion with smooth, fine wrinkles and a kind demeanor. He has a trim build and appears to be in excellent shape at age fifty-three. His uniform is typical battle dress and fits him well. He sits down towards one end of the long table and looks around the room. He is calm and collected, as if today is like any other day in Iraq.

The meeting begins with some general introductions of staff members, and then General Mattis gets down to business. He tells us we are going to take Fallujah, and anyone who threatens or opposes us will be eliminated, while those who cooperate will be rewarded and protected. The message he wants us to impress upon the Iraqi people is that we will be their friends if they help us, but we will be their worst enemy if they oppose us. The bulk of our battalion will be attacking the city from the south and the west of Fallujah. They will use superior fire power and air support to achieve victory. There are three battalions involved in the attack, and they will be coordinating their movements with ours. Bursts of adrenaline run through my veins. I have Skoal chewing tobacco in my lower lip and it adds to the rush. I feel like I'm living in a movie; lights from the projector flicker across Mattis's face as he describes the attack. Silhouettes of the company commanders outline the room, taking notes in their field books. Marines are the tip of the spear for ground offensives; the coordination of men and machinery is second to none. Upon conclusion of the meeting, General Mattis makes his orders clear: we will not stop until the city of Fallujah is ours.

Mattis concludes, then Captain Jamie Edge, the operations officer, gives more details about the operation. The attack on Fallujah had been brewing for days after Iraqi insurgents in Fallujah ambushed a convoy containing four American private military contractors from Blackwater USA. The four armed contractors, Scott Helvenston, Jerko Zovko, Wesley Batalona and Michael Teague, were killed by grenades thrown through the window of their armored vehicle. A mob set their bodies ablaze and their corpses were dragged through the streets before being hung over a bridge crossing the Euphrates. Crowds of young Iraqis swarmed below, chanting and yelling words of praise and triumph to Allah. These gruesome images were broadcast over and over around the world and, to many Americans, served as a compelling reminder of the level of hatred and evil of the insurgency. Fallujah, under the command of Abu Musab al-Zarqawi, remains a rising hotbed of anti-American activity and the source of terror for many Iraqi civilians. Al-Zarqawi is a rising star for the insurgents and quickly becoming responsible for multiple bombings, beheadings, and attacks. U.S. political leaders have decided that the city must be taken by force. The Marines will lead the charge with Navy medical support.

For tactical purposes, the city is divided into four quadrants, ideally with one battalion assigned to each one. However, only two assault battalions are available to initiate the attack. My battalion will lead the assault from the southeast portion of the city. Our Marines are equipped with night vision goggles and supported by AC-130 gunships for nighttime fighting. They will have additional air support from Air Force and Navy fighter jets loaded with laser-guided missiles and Cobra attack helicopters for daytime raids. Insurgents generally fight from hard points in buildings, only exposing themselves for seconds at a time. It is estimated there are up to twenty-four separate "hardcore" groups of insurgents, armed with rocket-propelled grenades (RPGs), machine guns, mortars, and anti-aircraft weapons in Fallujah. The Marines' primary approach is to isolate and destroy them by blockade of cross streets, then advance with tanks, air assets, and fire superiority.

The offensive is officially called Operation Vigilant Resolve; it is planned to be executed in four stages. Stage I involves a general cordon of Fallujah, vehicle check points, and blocking positions set up around the city. No one will be allowed to enter or leave. Anyone attempting to leave or break through the boundaries will be captured or killed. Stage II consists of tactical raids on high-value targets in Fallujah, to capture or kill personnel involved in attacks against coalition forces. Stage III includes the seizure of special objective points within the city known to harbor anti-coalition forces. Finally, stage IV consists of handing off combat operations to Iraqi security forces. Iraqi forces are integrated with Marine forces in each stage of the operation to emphasize the long-term goal of Iraqis establishing security and control of their country by their means. In all stages of the operation, the Marines will be conducting information operations

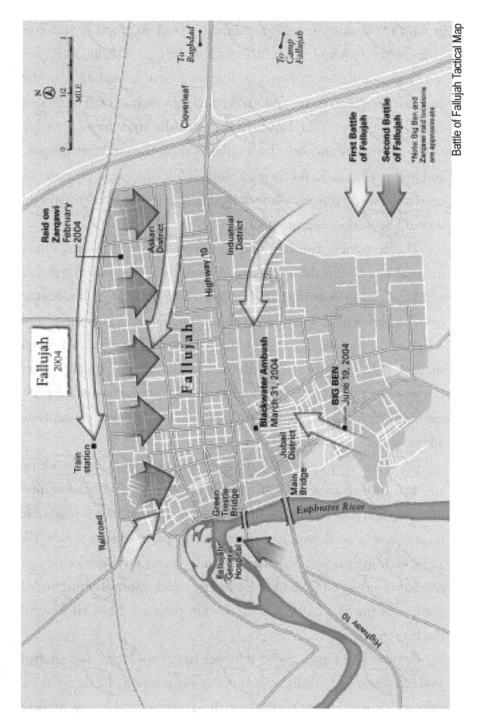

Battle of Fallujah Tactical Map

Fallujah 2004

Raid on Zarqawi February 2004

Cloverleaf

To Baghdad

To Camp Fallujah

First Battle of Fallujah

Second Battle of Fallujah

*Note: Big Ben and Zarqawi raid locations are approximate

Askari District

Industrial District

Highway 10

Fallujah

Blackwater Ambush March 31, 2004

BIG BEN June 19, 2004

Jubail District

Main Bridge

Green Trestle Bridge

Train station

Railroad

Euphrates River

Fallujah General Hospital

Highway 10

N

MILE

in which coalition messages are displayed and vocalized in order to gain cooperation and support from local citizens in Fallujah. There is a large population of Iraqis on the fence between siding with the enemy or coalition forces and we need to gain their trust. The goal of our message is two-fold: highlight the cowardly and deceptive nature of the insurgents and help Iraqi citizens to understand our purpose and intent as we fight for their freedom. With significant obstacles to overcome, we do not know how long this operation will take; I'm told it could be weeks, even months.

The corpsmen, Cormac, and I are tasked with providing direct medical support for the operation. We will be in position to stabilize and treat casualties as they are transported to us by ground medevac from the battlefield. Initially, command suggested that Cormac and I should be mobile, moving by ambulance or Humvee to injured marines in Fallujah for stabilization and treatment. We quickly point out our concerns for this plan and make the case for a forward positioned but stationary Battalion Aid Station, where we can concentrate all our medical capabilities.

Our Navy corpsmen are trained in tactical combat care, working side by side with infantry marines. Their role is to serve as an immediate medical provider in the field. There is no need, nor is it feasible for a doctor to be transported rapidly to the point of each injury. We argue each marine will be better served by temporary stabilization of combat injuries in the field, followed by rapid transportation out of the line of fire to a battlefield aid station positioned not far beyond the front lines.

Cormac and I anticipated that this issue could arise and studied evidence from past conflicts to support our position. There are three primary causes of death on the battlefield: severe head injury, massive bleeding, and collapsed lungs, also known as a tension pneumotho-rax. These causes of battlefield death have changed little since the first World War, and therefore all Navy corpsmen are trained to recognize and treat these wounds in the field. Military medicine has made minor advances in the initial treatment and stabilization of wounds in the field, but overall, the concepts have remained the same: stop the bleeding, protect the airway, and support breathing and cardiovascu-lar circulation. There is little that can be done in the field to treat a severe head wound, but the other two major causes of death can be adequately treated by a corpsman.

Massive bleeding can be controlled with pressure dressings, tour-niquets, and hemostatic agents, and a collapsed lung can be relieved by placing a large needle into the chest cavity to decompress the air surrounding the lung. Understandably, it can be difficult for military field commanders to accept that many combat injuries will result in death no matter how quickly they get to a doctor. Most battlefield deaths occur immediately or within the first five to ten minutes of an injury. The next group of patients who live beyond this point have significantly higher survival rates if they make it to a surgeon within one to two hours; therefore, we make the point to our commanding officer that if we establish a casualty collection point within five to ten minutes from the front lines, we can stabilize our marines here, then rapidly transport them to a surgical unit, well within an hour. Colonel Byrne voices comfort with our reasoning and we hammer out plans for the location of our forward BAS, the cloverleaf.

The cloverleaf is strategically ideal. Sitting just outside the Fallujah perimeter, with highway access and egress for rapid evacuation, it will serve the Marines well as they fight their way into the heart of Fallujah. When a Marine is injured in battle, the company corpsmen nearest to him will treat and stabilize him on scene, then load the Marine into a Humvee and transport him to us at the BAS, just a few minutes away. At the aid station we will continue stabilization and treatment of his wounds and then transfer him to an ambulance team who will transport him via armored convoy to the surgical company five miles away. If a wounded marine cannot be evacuated by ground, an air medevac will be requested by helicopter. This is the basic outline for our medical support of Operation Vigilant Resolve before the beginning of offensive actions. I am certain there will be many details and logistics that will change before the assault begins, and I prepare myself to remain flexible, as this is the Navy-Marine Corps way.

The bulk of our battalion leaves base on April 4th to establish battle positions and make final preparations for the offensive in Fallujah. Cormac leaves with the main body and seven corpsmen to set up the field BAS for medical support. I remain at Camp Mercury for now to provide medical care for Marines at the base and those injured in combat who have been sent back to Camp Mercury. I plan to meet up with Cormac at the cloverleaf in three to four days. My hope is that with the battalion gone it will be quiet for a while—I am very wrong.

It isn't hard to spot a huge convoy of marines leaving the base, and the insurgents keep a close eye for opportunity. Mortars start hitting the camp in the early morning of April 6th, continuing throughout the day into the night. I'm now able to estimate approximate distances of mortar impacts by the pitch and sound made when the blasts hit the ground. Distant mortars sound like muffled fireworks— bump-bump, bump…bump. Mortar impacts one to two kilometers away hit the ground with an uncomfortable crack, like lightning that makes you jump—*THWACK!* And mortars landing within half a kilometer or closer shake your bones and rattle your brain. No matter how common the attacks become, they still catch me off guard every time. They are merely a menace that poses a low risk of harm when landed outside the base walls, but the mental torment is brutal, lasting for short but intense periods. However, if they hit inside the walls, the outcome can be devastating.

Later that evening, I spend time at the COC listening to radio traffic about operations in Fallujah. Details are limited. The attack has begun and is making forward progress, but we are starting to take some casualties as the marines go building to building, clearing each block before moving on to the next. I recognize it's only a matter of time until some of our marines will be killed in action. I catch a few minutes of CNN on TV that night. The headlines are all about Fallujah and the chaos in the rest of Iraq; the Shias are rioting in Balad and the Iraqi Civil Defense Corps (ICDC) turned against coalition forces near Baghdad. General unrest is rampant, and the mood is all business at the COC. Since our arrival, the situation in Iraq has deteriorated; our call to action is perfectly timed, however I know it amounts to a heavy load for our men.

The next day, most of the battalion has pushed forward into Fallujah, and the compound feels empty. Mortars land sporadically throughout the day and night, just often enough to keep me on edge. Casualty reports drift in sporadically over the radio in the COC. Men are getting injured and even killed in Fallujah, and tensions are high. My daily report reads:

- Lance Corporal Marshall, shrapnel wounds to the upper body, stable condition, Alpha Company.

- Sergeant Pivin, gunshot wound to the left leg, serious injury and urgent medevac, Weapons Company.

- Private Stallworth, gunshot wound to the head, killed in action, Bravo Company.

I have the unforgiving job of tracking our casualties as the men are evacuated to various treatment facilities throughout Iraq. This is a painstaking and frustrating task, as communications between bases are fragile, and even when working, dropped calls are common. Commanders are always eager to know the status of their wounded men, and too often, I'm unable to provide the updates they want.

The offensive is now full tilt as I am backstage, restless and ready to move forward to assume my role in the assault unfolding in Fallujah. Transfer orders are handed down that night from headquarters; the next day I will board the first convoy leaving at dawn, and our first stop is the cloverleaf, Fallujah.

CHAPTER 7

The Cloverleaf,
April 8th, 2004 (+ 114)

"And I heard the voice of the Lord saying, 'Whom shall I send, and who will go for
us?' Then, I said, 'Here I am! Send me.'"

—*Isaiah, 6:8, English Standard*

We leave Camp Mercury for the cloverleaf in a convoy of seven trucks
at 10:00 a.m., and I'm sitting shotgun in a four-door Humvee. I'm
wearing my body armor; my head and face are fully covered with my
helmet, ballistic goggles, and nylon neck gator over mouth to keep the
dust out. My M9 pistol is strapped to my upper chest for easy access
with a right-hand grab. During the ride, it occurs to me if "the doctor"
ever needs to fire his weapon, things have gone wrong. Nevertheless,
I won't hesitate if the situation arises. Over my left shoulder, I see the
turret gunner's legs. He's standing upright, gripping his 50-caliber
machine gun. This formidable weapon is a welcome sight, boasting
a five-and-a-half inch cartridge with ample fire power; it is often the

choice for high-powered sniper rifles. Behind me are two Navy corpsmen with medical equipment and MRE boxes in the back. I'm edgy but pumped and ready to join my men at the BAS.

As the convoy lurches onto the main highway I notice a large faded green sign with white lettering hanging from the overpass ahead. The metal is twisted, rusted, and riddled with bullet holes. There is an arrow pointing straight ahead with the letters below spelling "Fallujah." It is mid-afternoon and already the winds are kicking up flurries of dust and sand that hang delicately in the air, obscuring the sun and creating a soft, sinister glow through the windshield. After a mile we roll into the cloverleaf at 11:00 a.m. The day is viciously hot; beads of sweat roll down the middle of my back as I step off the Humvee, planting my feet firmly on the hot pavement. I squint to see through the dusty breeze and adjust my Kevlar helmet to rest slightly tilted on my forehead, avoiding a small abrasion where the leather band has rubbed my skin raw. I scan the overpass as I walk from one side of the highway to the other; my desert brown boots lumber densely beneath the weight of my flak jacket and field gear. A scalpel, field dressings, and morphine hang from my vest, and now that I'm on site, I move my M9 to a thigh holster. I walk upright, chest out and chin up, attempting an outward appearance of confidence, knowing I am an unproven man entering a place that has seen turmoil and death.

To my right and left are dirt embankments leading up to the highway above us that runs east to west. Looking in this direction, I see only concrete columns and the cement underbelly of the highway overpass that provides a small semblance of protection. I climb the side of the eastern dirt embankment.

Looking two hundred yards down the road, I see marines have cordoned off passage into the cloverleaf. My eyes now turn to the south, and through the gritty orange haze I see more marines posted in Humvees mounted with heavy machine guns blocking another potential entrance to the cloverleaf. Their presence and fire power are formidable, and at about one hundred yards away, their silhouettes are reassuring. Standard issue is an M16 machine gun, while a few select men carry heavy 240 Golf or M249 Squad Automatic Weapon (SAW) machine guns.

I look to the north toward Fallujah. That town I read about, studied, and pictured over and over in my head as the months led up to our deployment. Television clips and aerial reconnaissance maps were the only images I knew until now. Staring at the outskirts of the city, the historical significance is not lost on me. Thirty-six miles west of Baghdad and I'm standing in the middle of the cradle of civilization, framed by the Tigris and Euphrates Rivers. It's hard to imagine, just a few miles south are the remains of the biblically important cities of Babylon and the Tower of Babel. At this moment, it feels like Hell.

I estimate the perimeter of the city to be four hundred yards away. I focus my eyes down the single-lane highway heading into Fallujah; it's like peering through a dirty window. The desert terrain along the highway is destitute of life. Near the city limits are buildings and homes with blown-out windows and wrecked vehicles abandoned on the side of the road. Soft ashen sand blows in loose swirls over the blacktop highway. Trash and tinder mingle about, tripping across the tortured earth. A wisp of hot wind whispers in my ear, giving way to a great sense of loneliness. I look for something of color and life as I gaze over the burnt-out wasteland, but there is nothing, only desolation and abandonment.

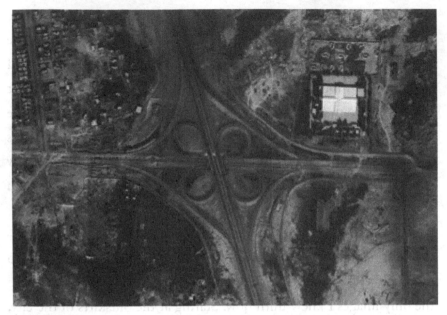

Aerial shot of Cloverleaf

The cloverleaf is a major route on the road from Baghdad to Fallujah, and therefore its occupation has been strategically important for both the insurgents and coalition forces throughout the Iraq War. For now, this cloverleaf will be my home, my office, my surgical unit, and the Battalion Aid Station.

As I walk towards the recently fabricated aid station, I see Cormac approaching me. He has been here for three days and I'm anxious to hear how things are going.

I throw down my field pack, and as we lock hands I say, "Hey brother, good to see you. How are you doing?"

He smiles and says, "Hey, Donnelly. I'm okay. Welcome to paradise, my friend."

Despite where we are, I manage to laugh and reply, "Haha, I brought my bathing suit. Which way is the swimming pool, next to the ammo depot?" We both laugh, then knowing time is precious, we get down to business.

"Okay, here is the situation. Captain Dickens and Charlie Company are in blocking position, cordoning off south of Fallujah. Captain Treglia and Alpha Company are north of the Euphrates river, pushing in from the southern flank of the city and making steady progress. We treated some Marines with gunshot and shrapnel wounds, and fortunately, all survived."

"How are Captain Smith and Bravo Company doing?" I ask.

"They have been in some heavy fire fights but are kicking ass," he says.

"Hell yes, I love it," I reply. "Okay, we brought more splints and morphine in the convoy, can you show me around?"

We walk towards the back of the Humvee ambulance while men offload fresh supplies, shout orders, and turn over duties to incoming personnel.

"We have all the medical supplies, trauma equipment, and medications positioned here and here," Cormac says as he points to each canister.

"How quickly can you get a ground medevac here?" I ask.

"From the time we radio headquarters, it takes about twenty minutes for them to arrive," he replies.

"How are the corpsmen doing? Are you guys taking any indirect fire?" I press.

"They are solid, but some could use a hot meal and shower. We got mortared a couple times last night, but no direct hits. Man, that will rock your sleep," he says, shaking his head.

"Yeah, we got hammered at the base the other night too. It's brutal," I say as I nod in agreement. Men behind us scurry into vehicles, taking their positions in the convoy as the trucks fire up engines to head for home base, Camp Mercury. I feel the need to ask important questions as our departure nears, knowing I'll be on my own soon without another physician to consult. I'm only able to blurt out one thought as Cormac grabs his gear and moves towards the vehicles. "Hey Cormac, can you email Katie in the next couple days to tell her I'm okay?"

"You bet, buddy, I'm on it, and I'll be monitoring your traffic on the radio!" he says loudly, over the roar of the engines as he climbs into an open-back Humvee.

"Okay brother, get some rest and watch some good flicks!" I scream back. He slides down ballistic goggles from his helmet over his eyes and gives me a thumbs-up as the convoy lurches forward like a locomotive.

Three days before my arrival at the cloverleaf, an advance party delivered essential supplies to operate our field Battalion Aid Station. Some of these are standardized field medical supplies called for by the Navy, while others are provisioning our medical team determined vital during planning for the offensive.

Preparing medical supplies for Fallujah felt like preparing to summit Everest. I only knew the basics and relied greatly on my guides, the Navy corpsmen. They are my right and left hands when mine are not available. They all have basic medical training, and some have more advanced skills as well. We share an uncompromised level of trust and move in synchrony from hours of training together in the field and hospital settings. Affectionately, the marines call the Navy corpsmen "Doc."

For field operations, we brought intravenous fluids, pressure dressings, surgical airway kits, oxygen, and chest tubes. Among the medications are antibiotics for infections or penetrating wounds, morphine for shrapnel and gunshot wounds, Imitrex for migraine headaches, and Valium for pain and anxiety after being wounded. We have spine boards, neck braces, arm slings, tourniquets, and quick-clot powder to help control massive bleeding. Our Humvee ambulance is loaded with stretchers, oxygen, water, band-aids, bullets, and enough food to last us for weeks. Despite the meticulous preparations, I still felt the daunting pressure of the task before me.

As the sound of the truck fades into the distance, I face the aid station that has now become my responsibility. A dry breeze blows dirt in my face as I wipe my mouth with my sleeve; for a moment, I digest the sights and sounds under the overpass. I know this place will soon challenge all my skills and mental strength. I know I will see men die and it leaves me with a sharp pain in my gut. Battlefield trauma, incoming mortars, combat stress—these certainties are all upon me now and haunt me as I take the measure of my confidence. Then, just as quickly as these thoughts appear, I shove them aside. Something inside helps me to do so. It's bigger than me, strangely reassuring and forcing me to focus at precisely the right time. There is no more room for deliberation, and now so little time to prepare for what is to come.

I approach Vasquez, one of our senior corpsmen, and we discuss how the last few days played out. He is a robust man with broad shoulders and a thick trunk. His dark, deeply set eyes hold stories of years in the Navy and numerous deployments. His face has thick skin with contoured wrinkles around his mouth and forehead. I trust him and know he can provide me with direction in a combat environment. In turn, he looks to me for medical expertise and help making decisions, and thus we carry on a battlefield tradition that has endured for centuries between officer and enlisted personnel.

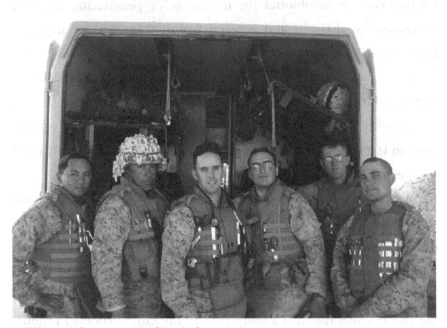

Lt. Wilkes with Corpsmen at the Cloverleaf

He briefs me on the layout of the aid station. The triage and treatment areas are positioned off to one side of the road, directly under the overpass for protection. Three litter stands are positioned in the gravel just off the pavement. Each has a green metal canister at the head, prepped and ready for trauma. To the left of the litter stands are steel and mesh lined barriers filled with dirt to protect from indirect gunfire and incoming mortars. At the heads of the stretchers are folding tables and silver metal cans piled with bandages, gauze, oxygen canisters, antibiotics, syringes, cervical collars, and leg splints.

I bend down at the head of a stretcher with one knee in the gravel. I pick through each item, turning them over in my hands as I hold them. I review instructions on surgical airways kits, flick on switches to headlamps and battery-powered laryngoscopes, and play out trauma scenarios in my head. I look out at the desert as sweat drips from my brow onto the ground, creating little puffs of dust with each drop.

After some time, I decide to rest, and so I sit down on the back of our ambulance. I breathe in the thick, grainy air; the taste of it lingers in my mouth. My armored flak jacket digs into my shoulders as I struggle to get comfortable sitting on the steel ambulance bumper. My chest heaves up and down underneath the weight of my jacket and my thoughts wander. My life's work will mean nothing if I can't put it all together now. Four years of college, one year of post-graduate school, four years of medical school, a one-year internship, officer indoctrination training, combat trauma training, and many hours of field training in the military—it all might come down to a single moment, and it weighs heavily on me now.

I look up and stare at the walls of Fallujah. It is not far down the road. I debate if there are snipers in the distance planning and spying on us, to position themselves for just the right shot. Could they hit us with an AK-47 from that distance, or mortars, or perhaps a rocket-propelled grenade? Without a good reason, I conclude these events are unlikely, and I feel more at ease for the moment. I turn around and look in the other direction.

About a half mile away I see what appears to be a large factory. I ask one of the marines if anyone has cleared these buildings. He tells me it is an abandoned glass plant and it is not a threat. With skeptical resignation, I turn back around and do not say anything. I look down at the ground. A parade of black ants races past my boots in a panic about something. A few minutes pass by. I stare at my watch, looking at the seconds tick by, and then look back up at my home under the highway overpass. This is my first hour at the cloverleaf.

At this stage of the offensive, U.S. forces from First Marine Division have cordoned off all routes into and out of the cloverleaf. Marines block all roads leading into the city with concertina wire and Humvees armed with fifty caliber machine guns and grenade launchers.

Marines took over a local radio station and handed out leaflets urging residents to remain inside their homes or vacate the city. Residents are urged to help American forces identify insurgents or any Fallujans involved in the deaths of the Blackwater contractors. The heart of the attack is aimed at isolating and rooting out insurgent forces responsible for repeated attacks on coalition forces to seize control of the city.

The first three days of fighting have been brutal but successful. Ground forces attacked from multiple directions, conducting close-quarter fights to sweep through a labyrinth of buildings and homes. Jihadi fighters had spent nearly six months constructing bunkers, choke points, ambushes, and avenues of retreat. Entire homes have been booby-trapped, streets and alleys have been laden with IEDs and blockades of rubble or junked cars. Every approach is expertly rigged with deadly hazards. U.S. forces are undeterred. Air strikes rain down on insurgent strongholds. F-18 Hornet fighter jets from the *USS George Washington* in the Arabian Gulf lay down twenty-millimeter cannons on enemy positions. Humvee-mounted TOW missiles are unleashed. These tube-launched, optically-tracked, wire-guided missiles can pound through barricades and armored vehicles with awesome accuracy. United States Air Force AC-130 Spectre gunships hit the enemy with incredible lethality, their Gatling guns and howitzers pounding insurgent positions. Captain Treglia and Alpha

Company are pushing in from thesoutheast flank while Captain Sokol and Weapons Company support the attack with heavy gun-trucks and mobile assault platoons. Snipers pick off targets from rooftop positions as our marine platoons fight relentlessly from building to building, clearing each block methodically before moving to the next.

Now it's my turn to take a front seat near Fallujah. For a few hours, I walk through our BAS, reviewing our capabilities, supplies, and the limited protection we have under the overpass. I keep close contact with my corpsmen, checking their gear, and asking how they're doing. I review communications with our Marines protecting the perimeter access points into the cloverleaf, confirming our tactical position under the overpass is sound.

Corpsman Aircroth monitors the radio, providing updates on the assault. Vasquez and I review our medical supplies, ensuring we have our equipment prepped and ready. Finally, I'm satisfied with my walk-through and confident we're prepared. I'm feeling focused and poised. I'm locked on my mission and ready to do my duty. I walk to the edge of the road, stepping onto the pavement I pat my M9 pistol, adjust my flak and helmet, turn my eyes west towards Fallujah, and earnestly wait for action.

A FALLEN LEAF

BAP, BAP, BAP! Blum, boom-boom! My head jerks up and my eyes ratchet forward. I'm standing under the overpass when I hear an unsettling popping thunder five hundred yards in front of me. I focus on the perimeter buildings of Fallujah in the direction of the blasts, as black mist seeps into the air above the rooftops like a signal marking death. Eyesight narrows and leg muscles tighten. Tiny beads of perspiration crowd my forehead as I anticipate what happens next. "Here we go," I think.

Minutes later I hear the high-powered winding of engines in the distance, like a wounded animal giving away its location. I peer down the road to see a Humvee roaring towards us with dust clouds and dirt spewing behind it, a sense of urgency in its approach. With dread I know there must be wounded men on board. They come up on us fast, a corpsman steps out onto the road with both hands held high, sweeping his arms down and to the left, towards our treatment area. The Humvee screeches to a halt in front of our litter stands; dust clouds and diesel fumes fill the air.

As they open the back of the Humvee, I yell for a stretcher. The closest one is next to me, littered with medical supplies. I motion for it, and in one fell swoop, Aircroth wipes it clean with his arms, sending boxes of supplies flying. Four marines jump out of the back and pull a limp body from the bed of the vehicle. My heart sinks as I see the gunshot wound to the back of his head. Fellow marines lift him onto the stretcher on the ground and continue to yell desperate words of encouragement to their fallen brother. "Keep breathing, Jackson, don't give up!"

Enter Navy medical. Field medicine is vastly different from hospital medicine. Under any normal circumstances, you have time to order studies to help make decisions—things like labs, scans, and diagnostics. Advanced monitoring and imaging can help to assess cardiac and lung conditions before interventions are made. Blood tests may yield insight into a problem before it gets worse. In the field, you only have the tools you brought with you and your clinical skills. Decisions must be made quickly, sometimes on the fly without the diagnostic tools you're used to. If you make a mistake, even one that causes harm, you must forgive it and move on—there is no time for remorse. All the marines want to know is that you'll do absolutely everything you can. The environment is unforgiving; lighting is poor, the heat intense, and working conditions harsh on the ground. Add combat to the mix and it's like ballet with a bull.

We clear the area, kneel next to Lieutenant Jackson, and go to work. I'm at his head while our corpsmen are scattered around his body. His condition is critical from the start. He has a massive head wound with brain matter protruding from the frontal portion of his skull. Flecks of dried blood speckle his face and sweat mixed with dirt stains his body.

"Put a moist gauze over his head wound," I say while trying to sort out the situation.

His skin is ashen and his pupils are sluggish. He is barely breathing on his own and we immediately decide to attempt an intubation. We've got to get him oxygen quickly. My thoughts race. "Lord, how is this man still alive?" His injury is almost certainly a mortal wound.

I shout above the commotion, "I need an intubation kit and light!" I know it will be a desperate and extremely difficult procedure to perform on the ground, with poor lighting and no way to elevate his body. Even if we are successful in stabilizing him, I know the odds of his survival with any meaningful recovery are horribly dim. I am painfully aware that his fellow marines look on directly behind me. Some of them continue to shout from the sidelines, while others stare at us with blank hopelessness. Their presence alone confirms my resolve to do everything humanly possible for this marine. We cannot let them believe for one moment that we will do anything less for each one of them. Part of the marines' unrelenting resolve is the knowledge they will have the best medical care possible if they are injured, and I know we need to prove this to them now. And so, the effort continues as we work on the ground in the dirt and in the wind. Men move around us, some looking, some not daring to.

"We need to get this tube in now," I say, knowing the seconds are critical. My knees grind on the ground and my heart heaves beneath my vest while my hands try to move fast. Bombs explode and gunfire echoes in the background.

I attempt to intubate three times, carefully directing the breathing tube down his throat into his trachea, the main airway. Each one is unsuccessful, just missing the main entry point. Between attempts, I continue to provide artificial breathing for him with a bag and mask over his face. I sweat and breathe faster in my flak jacket; I wish we weren't working on the ground in the suffocating heat. Corpsmen shout out vital signs and I see that he is fading.

"His breathing is shallow and his blood pressure is dropping," I say.

"Should we try a cricothyroidotomy?" I say to myself. "Yep, let's do it," I reply within seconds.

A cricothyroidotomy is a surgical procedure in which a small incision is made into the membrane of the main airway, near the Adam's apple of the neck. Then, a stylet is used to widen the hole, and an airway tube is inserted. Next, a small balloon is inflated to seal the airway around the tube, and finally, a tube is attached to a bag you squeeze to provide ventilation into the lungs. It is a difficult procedure to perform under these circumstances, but we know it's our only hope to secure his airway. The first attempt fails. *Focus now,* I think.

The second time is successful. I hook up the bag-valve-mask to the breathing tube and give respirations. One-two-three, breathe. One-two-three, breathe. I watch his chest artificially rise and fall as I squeeze the bag. Chief Vasquez checks his pulse—nothing. He isn't responding. I hear gunfire in the distance and a helicopter as it flies overhead. I keep squeezing that damn bag. A few painful minutes go by. He has no pulse and no breath. He is killed in action. Vasquez's eyes meet mine and we nod.

"All right, everyone, let's stop resuscitative efforts. He's gone," I say.

There are no words for a long minute, and I contemplate what to do next. There is no training for this moment, and nothing seems sufficient. I look around in front of me, then to my left and right. There are seven of us, kneeling on the ground and huddled over our marine.

Slowly, each of us release ourselves from the moment as our muscles relax and we lean back on our heels like a tire losing air. I turn around to see silent eyes on the faces of tired and war-torn marines. I struggle for a single word. A string of sweat runs down my spine as I look at our dead marine. I am lost for a moment, but then I know what to do.

"Okay guys, everyone gather around him," I say. We encircle his body; each man links arms to the next. My voice cracks when I first open my mouth, I pause, and then firmly say, "Lord, we kneel here together with our fallen brother. We can't fully understand his death and our grief that will follow. We lift him up to you and pray for mercy and healing for his family. We pray for courage, righteous victory, and the strength to go on in this fight as brothers in Christ, Amen."

I kneel with one hand on the ground and the other on my head. Some men cry. I stand up and look around under the highway overpass. Everything is still. There are bloody bandages, IV tubing, and spent medical supplies strewn everywhere. His helmet and M16 still lie next to him with blood on the ground, mixed in the dirt. His brown flak jacket is folded next to him and I pick it up. It has a bullet hole in it, from which we pull out a twisted hunk of metal—the remnants of the bullet that went into his chest.

Bombs and bullets continue to ring in the background and smoke spirals upward from the homes in Fallujah. On the embankment to my left, I see his company senior marine sitting with his face buried in his hands and he is in tears. It's the singular moment every commander dreads.

For a minute, my thoughts drift to how my path led me to this place, witnessing this magnitude of death; it is more than I expected. When I joined the Navy before medical school, it was peacetime. The possibility of embarking with an infantry battalion to combat was never even mentioned. After 9/11, all of this changed. Tranquil Pacific fleet deployments became Middle East combat deployments.

All non-military doctors complete three to five years of residency training before practicing medicine autonomously. This is not the case for military doctors. As it was for me, we can be pulled from residency after the first year of training (internship) and deployed for active duty, piling an immense level of responsibility on a young physician. During my field medical training, I came to understand this responsibility and accept it—now I'm feeling the weight of it. (This rule has since changed, requiring all physicians to complete full residency training before embarking on active duty assignments.)

I feel so far away from the small northern California town where I grew up. The life I knew, summer days spent working with my four brothers in the gardens and orchards of our five acres in the foothills of the Sierra Nevada mountains. Weekends and summers playing baseball in the local town league, laboring at my father's construction sites, and coming home to my mother's kind voice and home cooking. All of this feels so foreign to me now; it is distressingly distant and tugs at my emotions. I'm on the other side of the world and it feels like I'll never get back.

I shake my head back to reality, get up off my knees, and again break the silence, shouting, "Okay, let's get this place cleaned up and get ready for more casualties!"

As my corpsmen prepare the aid station, I hear a convoy steam into the overpass. Expecting the worst, I walk briskly towards the lead Humvee parked next to the stretchers. Then I see Captain Phil Treglia exit the vehicle and turn in my direction. He's walking fast, spots me and dons a familiar smile. He is dirty from head to toe, like he just surfaced from a coal mine. At six-one and two hundred eight pounds, Phil is a heavy hitter. He is Caucasian with brownish-red hair, blue eyes, and a deep voice. Born and raised in Elida, Ohio, his father was a marine and he followed suit. He attended Ohio State University on a Marine Corps scholarship and graduated officer candidate school with honors. As a veteran of Afghanistan and a specialist in night raids, he is the perfect company commander for urban combat in Fallujah. We greet each other enthusiastically, grabbing hands and pulling in close for a quick chest bump.

"Hey brother, how are you guys holding up?" he says.

"Hey buddy, we're doing our best, receiving some serious casualties," I say.

"We've got your back, you just stay strong," he replies.

"I've heard some intense fighting from here; how are your marines?" I ask.

"Rattled, but strong. We took some serious small-arms fire and RPGs as the company attacked across phase line violet (front line of the battle), but only one wounded in action," he states.

"Ok man, I love it. We're standing by if you need anything," I reply.

Despite his war face Phil is energetic, confident, and even excited. Is it possible he feels as good as he sounds? Then it occurs to me, he's in his element. He's a warrior, strapped from head to toe, and right where he wants to be. I'm inspired and fired up at the sight of his resilience. My spirits lift just knowing Phil and his marines are in Fallujah laying down heavy fire to protect us, driving back the enemy. He stays for a short time to plan his egress and gather supplies, then storms out as quickly as he arrived.

One week later a photograph of us praying over our marine on bended knees made the front page of the *New York Times* and *Washington Post*. Since then, this Pulitzer Prize-winning picture has been featured in news magazines, posters, and circulated in numerous email chains.

At the time this picture was taken, and unknown to me, an *Associated Press* photographer named Murad Sezer was posted at the cloverleaf. He had been dropped off at our position and was waiting for a convoy out of the cloverleaf the same day our marine was killed. He witnessed all that happened that day under the overpass as we worked and prayed over him, and then he captured its finality in a photograph.

Before the photographer leaves the cloverleaf that day, he approaches me and says, "Until today I have never seen a man die before."

"It's a very sobering and humbling experience, isn't it?" I reply.

"I can't find the words to describe it," he responds.

"I know what you mean. I feel that way about a lot of the things I've seen here," I say.

He pauses then says, "I think the most agonizing and perhaps helpless part of what I saw was when you and your men were hud-

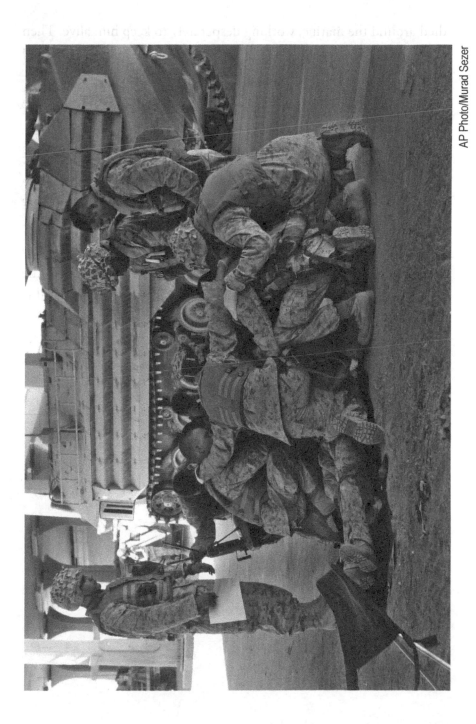

AP Photo/Murad Sezer

dled around the marine, working desperately to keep him alive. Then when you knew he had died, you gave the word, and everyone leaned back on their knees, all at the same time, sort of in defeat."

I nod slowly as the scene comes back to me, but I say nothing. He wishes me well, then we shake hands and he walks away.

Until then, I hadn't considered what it looks like from the sidelines to watch a struggle for life end in defeat. Particularly, I thought, for someone outside the military and the Marine Corps. Following my deployment, as the years pass and my life unfolds, this photograph finds its way to me, as both a picture and a memory etched into my soul. It haunts me, humbles me, and I still catch my breath as the sadness creeps in, remembering all that happened on this memorable day at the cloverleaf.

CHAPTER 8

The Spiritual Reckoning

I did not know at the time that my spiritual reckoning would meet me at the cloverleaf. I did not know it would help me endure, yet it did. I did not foresee it would give me strength, but it did. And I could not see that it would change my heart, although it would. It happened on the night Lieutenant Jackson died, after my first day at the cloverleaf, April 8th, 2004. That's the day we all tried our best, while others watched, yet it ended in defeat. We put his body in a black bag, the kind with the long zipper. He was taken away in an armed escort and we stared as they drove out of sight. It was on this night in the back of my ambulance, sorting through the pieces of a life lost, in the middle of Iraq, that my life came full circle. The events of that first night come back to me now clearly, like a scent you can't erase, like a light that never burns out, each time I return to that night of nights.

Sitting in the back of my Humvee ambulance, I peer through a crack in the steel double doors; I can see the outline of medical equipment and stretchers in the dark. Beyond these silhouettes, faint lights speckle the outskirts of Fallujah. I lie down, trying to sleep; the other men have gone to bed and I'm alone with my thoughts. Images of war flash through my head, mixed with longing thoughts of home. "*This place is surreal; how will I describe it to my family?*" I think. Outside the ambulance, Humvees, tanks, and other assault vehicles rumble by from time to time. The ambulance shakes and dust floats down upon my head as they drive by. I place foam plugs in my ears, attempting to dampen the noise, but they are comically ineffective. I wriggle down into my standard-issue green sleeping bag, struggling to get comfortable on the nylon stretcher. The handles on the sides poke into my ribs. I pore over the day's events over and over, picturing Lieutenant Jackson lying on the ground, the bullet in his flak jacket, the desperation in the eyes of his friends. Somewhere amid these thoughts, I drift off to sleep.

A few hours pass and suddenly my eyes pop wide open. It takes me a moment to figure out why, then I hear the hard popping of machine guns. The gunfire is from Fallujah, and I gently twitch on my rack as the fire fight carries on. There is a pause, long enough for my muscles to relax and my shoulders to sink back into the mesh of the stretcher, then suddenly incoming rounds pound the ground outside. The ambulance cage shakes, my body jerks upward as my hands cover my head. My heart races and fear clouds my brain. Anxious and trapped in my steel tomb, I begin to spiral into thought. "*What I should do? Should I put on my flak jacket? Are more wounded men on the way?*" I breathe faster, my heart pumps in my chest and in my ears. I think about Katie and home, but they are so distant, like a familiar dream I can't remember. Tears of frustration well in my eyes; I want it all to go away. I start asking God some serious questions.

"*Why the hell have you brought me here? This isn't what I expected and this isn't what I thought you had planned for my life! Why me, God?*"

I stare intensely into the darkness consuming me inside my green prison. I can't see any rational end to my situation. The future is a black hole that means nothing to me; I feel the weight of my predicament crushing me. I have always been a person of inner strength and self-reliance; now I feel my confidence slipping from my hands. Right outside my door other men face their demons, many have it much worse, but it doesn't matter, my fear tells me; I'm on my own and I believe it. The burden is mine to bear, each mortar blast drives my loneliness deeper into my heart, each gunshot echoes my distance from home, and each wounded man is a sobering testament to the fragility of life. My fear is the enemy. I can't fight back, it has control over my life and death, and it's winning.

Feeling my frustration reaching a boiling point, I bury my face in my hands, crying in silent screams. I need to get control of my emotions or they will ruin me, but how? I am lost, wasting away, and I know it. I start to pray, as I have done many days before, but this time I sense something has to be different. I'm holding on too tight, praying desperately for a release. "*Yes…maybe that's it,*" I think, "*a final release is what I long for, but how?*"

"*I have done everything asked of me,*" I think. I prepared physically, mentally, and logistically for my mission, yet here I am, lost and struggling for answers. I knew this place might be hell, but I thought I could handle it better.

Then a question hits me right between the eyes: Why do you insist on shouldering this burden on your own? Don't you know God promised He will never leave you, that He is asking you to release your pain and fear to Him? I pause for a moment to think, "*Is it that simple, is this message really for me?*" And then God's promise comes flooding back to me like a warm memory and I know what I need to do. I climb from my rack onto my knees in the back of the ambulance. I feel the cold steel and hard grains of dirt against my kneecaps, and for the first time in many days, I sense a tide is about to turn. I begin to pray. It's simple, but my heart is different.

"Lord, I am lost and confused, I've refused to accept my fate—to be persecuted with bombings and an attendant to death. I know you have a reason beyond my understanding why you brought me to this place. All my life I've listened to your teachings and lived by your word, but no matter how I've tried, I never released control of my life to you. Today is just another example of my desperate struggle, pretending I can handle it on my own. Please help me now. Lord, I release the last threads of control over my life to you. My fears of failure, loneliness, and death—I give them all to you. Release my weakness, transform me with your grace and strength. With you, I cannot fail."

I rise from my knees a new man in Christ, accepting and believing why God brought me to the cloverleaf: to sever the final threads of control.

"*Then so be it, I will do whatever is asked of me,*" I vow then and there. I know it's what must be done for me to make it through.

I feel the weight lifting from my shoulders, understanding my trials are not miraculously ending and many still lie ahead, but that victory is closer than ever and fear no longer has hold over me. I know God will not leave me, in life or in death, and no matter what the outcome of today or any other day, I cannot be defeated with God's grace. It is a strength I have not felt in a long time, a strength that assures me of God's love in times of doubt, fear, and even death, knowing I am never alone.

CHAPTER 9

The Cloverleaf, Day Two, April 9th, 2004 (+ 115)

At 7:00 a.m., I wake to the sound of vehicles passing through the cloverleaf, intrusive and raucous. The ground quakes as they pass. It is cold in the back of the ambulance that morning. Still half asleep, I duck my head back into my down sleeping bag as I slowly regain consciousness of the previous twenty-four hours. "*Okay, I'm in Iraq, in the back of an ambulance, under a highway…this is the beginning of my second day at the cloverleaf, that's right.*"

I swear I have already been there for days, but reality tells me the truth. My back aches, and I squirm to get comfortable on my stretcher. My arm is numb from sleeping on the poles suspending the nylon mesh that keeps me folded like a taco. Time seems to be moving in sections, painfully and slowly. Activity hummed along the cloverleaf all night and I did not sleep well. Humvees, tanks, seven-ton trucks, and amphibious assault vehicles hammered at the walls of the overpass throughout the night, rumbling through determined and strong. In a strange way, it is comforting to know I sleep among these masses of mechanized, battle-ready steel, but it makes consistent sleep very difficult. This morning, an F-18 Hornet dropped two 500-pound laser-guided bombs on insurgent strongholds. The massive explosion rattled through the cloverleaf like a buffalo stampede.

Images of war and wounded marines crowd my thoughts. I remember Lieutenant Jackson, the marine we tried to save, and I wonder if there is more we could have done. Is there something we forgot, anything that could have made a difference? This is a ritual I sometimes torment myself with. It keeps me from becoming over-confident, but it also incites speculation and doubt. I know very well nothing could have saved this young man's life—he had a mortal head wound. Despite this, I persist in the mental gymnastics, and then my thoughts shift to home, to Katie, and my family. How will I explain this to them, this horrible place and the sadness that lives here? I suspect I cannot, that words will be insufficient, and that only to see it, feel it, and live it can explain what I know.

As I lie there in my rack, my covers up to my eyes, fending off the day, these thoughts pile on each other and I feel the creep of despair setting in. It's an insidious feeling of desolation, realizing what lies ahead, day after day, to earn the right to go home. It's intimidating, but I know I can endure, reminding myself I have the tools and skills for the job. Despite the intimidation, I'm driven to my duty, like a fireman to a fire. I've been handed the baton, and now it's my turn to run. I throw off the covers and breathe warm air into my hands. My spirits steadily lift and I move forward. I swing my legs over the stretcher onto the cold, dirty floor, then grab some baby wipes to clean my feet, underarms, and hands. I smell cleaner, but this process only seems to move the dirt around my body rather than remove it. I pull my green fleece sweater over my head, put on my desert camouflage pants, a new pair of black wool socks, and lace up my boots. My underwear will have to last another day.

As I push open the back double doors of the ambulance, the morning sun hits my eyes. I squint and sneeze once before I step out. I grab my hygiene bag, a bottle of water, and climb down the stepladder. Everyone is up and moving, except for one marine lying on the gravel next to the ambulance in his sleeping bag. I step around him, careful not to disturb his sleep, then proceed to the designated dirt latrine.

As I splash cold water on my face from my water bottle, I pause and glance upward at the outskirts of Fallujah. It is right in front of me, staring at me; nothing moves or even smiles. I marvel at the uniformity of brown that consumes the view—the ground, the dust-coated plants, hard crusts of earth, pasty brown buildings, the air—everything. Even the dirt looks dirty. I continue brushing my teeth with one eye on Fallujah. I opt for a speedy electric shave while peering into the side-view mirror of the ambulance. Finally, I strap on my flak jacket, helmet, and pistol before walking across the black pavement, over the center divider, and across the other side of the highway to greet the other men for an MRE breakfast. Lieutenant O'Connor rejoined us late yesterday on a supply convoy. Due to the intensity of combat in Fallujah and expected casualties, command agreed he should be with me at the cloverleaf rather than the BAS at Camp Mercury. They are standing just off the pavement in the dirt, eating, talking, and making plans for the day. I gladly join the circle.

At 10:00 a.m., word comes over the radio that two casualties are coming in by ground evac. Their injury status is unknown. Five minutes later, the Humvees storm into the cloverleaf. They know exactly where to stop. Engines rev, exhaust fills the air, and large tires screech to a halt. Corpsmen haul two marines onto stretchers from the back of the vehicle—both are seriously injured. One has a gunshot wound to the throat, and the other has a gunshot wound to his right thigh. Cormac takes charge of the first marine, Sergeant Morton, while I take the second, Corporal Bradley. We know they will both need a surgeon as soon as possible, and we immediately order our radioman to call for an urgent medical evacuation by ground. While we wait for the convoy to arrive, we commence with all-out efforts to stabilize the injured men.

Two corpsmen carry Corporal Bradley onto a stretcher from the back of the Humvee to a litter stand in front of me. While I quickly survey his injuries, they go to work cutting off his cammies, placing IVs in both arms, and administering oxygen. He has an in-and-out gunshot wound to his right thigh. The bleeding appears to be minimal, but he is going in and out of consciousness and not answering my questions accurately. I ask my corpsman for his vital signs. His pulse rate is normal, but his breathing is rapid and his blood pressure is low. His fingers are cold and clammy and turning blue. He is in shock, but whether emotional or traumatic shock I cannot tell. I look closer at the gunshot wound again. There is a pinkish-red opening in the middle of his thigh and what looks like an exit wound a few centimeters away.

The flesh is ripped, with jagged edges and charred black skin. There is no way I can tell if the bullet has penetrated deeper or not. His boots are still strapped on tightly, so I can't check for pulses in his feet; Vasquez is struggling to get them off. There's not an obvious deformity of his leg to imply a femur fracture, but it is very swollen where the bullet has entered. Although I feel it's unlikely, I must consider that his tenuous vital signs are due to hemorrhagic shock.

Without knowing the path of that bullet, I determine he may have an injury to his femoral artery, which can cause severe blood loss. I tell my corpsmen to begin infusing fluids rapidly into large-caliber IVs. We place a splint along his thigh and a large pressure dressing wrap over the bullet wound. My attention now turns to his face. He is ashen with wandering eyes, so I prop his head in my palm and shake him for a response. His eyes turn to me as he says, "Sir, I'm in a lot of pain"—a good sign showing he is alert enough to recognize his pain and tell me about it. After fluids have been running for a few minutes, he begins to come around and his blood pressure rises. I give him ten milligrams of morphine by intramuscular injection into his uninjured thigh. A few minutes pass and he tells me the pain is less. He is now breathing slower, and the color changes to pink in his fingers. He is stable, but I want to get him on an ambulance to the surgical company as soon as possible.

I turn to my left. Doctor O'Connor is struggling with Sergeant Morton right next to me, so I move in to offer help. His injuries are much more dire. He has a gunshot wound to the neck with an exit wound in his upper back. He is in critical condition upon arrival and very combative. It takes five men to hold him down enough to help him. Cormac has stabilized his airway and pushed IV fluids; initially, it seems his condition is improving, but shortly after, he takes a turn for the worse. His blood pressure drops and his pulse is racing. We place a needle into his upper chest cavity to see if there is air trapped around his lungs that is suffocating him. The needle decompression does not help. Cormac feels he likely has internal bleeding around his lungs and needs a chest tube urgently to drain the blood and ease his breathing. I agree, and we rapidly prep for a chest tube placement.

The ambulance convoy arrives for immediate evacuation to the surgical company. We load our marines in the back, and Cormac jumps in with them. He plans to place a chest tube while driving to the surgical company. Both of us know this will be a difficult, last-ditch effort to save the Sergeant's life, but we also know it is the right thing to do. We close the doors to the ambulance, give the driver a thumbs up, and they speed away. The armored security vehicles follow closely behind.

I turn around to look at the mess of medical equipment and trash strewn everywhere. Still breathing heavy with sweat dripping from my brow, I yell to the corpsmen to get the area cleaned up and ready for more casualties. Before they can even begin, another Humvee comes tearing down the road and brakes hard to stop right in front of us. A distraught appearing marine jumps out from the passenger side and yells, "Help us! I think our Sergeant is dead!" From the back of the vehicle, two men grab his shoulders, while two others grab his legs, and they all proceed to pull a very lifeless marine from the Humvee, then place him on a stretcher on the side of the road. He is young and tall, in his twenties, clean shaven with tightly trimmed hair. I kneel next to him, placing the bell of my stethoscope over his heart to look for signs of life—a breath, a pulse, a reactive pupil—but there is nothing.

A crowd of marines stands over me, patiently waiting for the outcome. His pupils are fixed straight ahead, dilated wide open and dark. He has no pulse or lung sounds. He is dead, killed in action in Fallujah. I give the word and we gather around him in prayer. Stillness is all around, haze and murk, metal and fear. I start to talk but then pause. My tear ducts open, but I squeeze tightly and clench my eyes. I cannot show my emotions at this moment; it is not the appropriate time and there will be occasion for this on another day. The men stand beside me and around me as I continue to speak over the dead marine. It is short and to the point; I pray for his family, strength, healing, and victory.

I stand up, looking around his body. His blood-stained uniform and used medical supplies are strewn about in the dirt. A flak jacket and M16 still lie next to him. His vest has a hole in it. We dislodge a piece of metal casing, evidence of his fate. In the near distance, I can hear attack helicopters and bullets piercing the evening air. Smoke billows from buildings in the background, some of them just a few hundred meters away. Chills wriggle down my spine and gnawing anger fills my heart. "So, this is war," I think. It is everything and nothing like I thought it would be.

CHAPTER 10

The Cloverleaf, Day Three, April 10th, 2004 (+ 116)

Gunfire and violence dominate the streets of Fallujah late into the night. As I huddle down inside the ambulance, falling in and out of sleep, I listen to the orchestra of munitions echo in the distance. I know it's close, but how close is what keeps me awake. *Grrr, rum, BAP*; grenades rumble and machine guns pop. I used to flinch and jerk with the sound of each blast, but now I only blink hard and clench my jaw, as if attempting to shake a terrible thought from entering my brain. My corpsmen taught me how to recognize different types of machine guns and artillery by the distinct sounds they make. It's a game I play to pass the time, trying to convince myself the explosions are farther off than I know they are.

There are others beyond the cloverleaf, directly in harm's way, unable to retreat to safer grounds. They are the warriors I am here to support—the Marines and Navy corpsmen of the 1st Marine Division. This is my focus and my mission, and it not only helps me stay motivated to remember my calling but also helps me find respite as I lie in my rack listening to the chaotic chorus in Fallujah. My mind drifts and I fall in and out of sleep; it's enough to get through the night, and I wake just before dawn as an amphibious assault vehicle tumbles my canteen and M9 pistol on the floor next to me. I roll off the cot, pull on my boots, strap on my flak, helmet, pistol, and I'm ready for the day—nothing to it.

The day prior, I learned coalition forces had unilaterally called a ceasefire among the Iraqi governing council, insurgents, and city spokespersons to allow government supplies to be delivered to residents. This allows Fallujah General Hospital to reopen for humanitarian relief necessitated by the fighting within the city and gives residents time to tend to the wounded and dead, but unfortunately, it also allows insurgents time to regroup and reinforce their positions. Hundreds of insurgents have been killed in the assault, and U.S. forces have only managed to gain a stronghold in the southern industrial district of Fallujah, and deep into the city from the north. Despite this, the insurgency remains dug-in throughout many sectors of Fallujah. Sporadic fighting continues throughout the city, and it is easy to forget that a so-called ceasefire is actually in place.

At 9:00 a.m., a large crowd of Iraqi protestors gathers at the east end of the cloverleaf. They have been displaced from their homes due to the battle in Fallujah, and now they want back into the city. Many of them have family or friends who unwisely decided to stay in the city and now are enduring the consequences. Members of the U.S.-appointed Iraqi Governing Council are strongly criticizing the U.S. military over civilian casualties, insisting the military response in Fallujah is overwhelming and indiscriminate. U.S. military spokesman Brigadier General Mark Kimmitt reports insurgents in the city are using Iraqi civilians as human shields and firing weapons at U.S.

forces from inside schools, mosques, and hospitals. As expected, they are ignoring the traditional covenants of war.

The protestors have come by the hundreds on foot and in cars, carrying signs and chanting. From our position, we can see a restless mob coalescing down the highway, only a few hundred yards away. Our concern is that this crowd may rapidly turn hostile and attack our position if tensions escalate. Shortly after their arrival, twenty to thirty troops and armored vehicles roar past us to control the situation. They roll out concertina wire and set up a perimeter to keep the crowds from advancing. Someone from the crowd manages to fire an RPG directly down the highway towards the cloverleaf. It sputters to a halt fifty yards from our position without exploding—a dud. We snap pictures of it like it's a tourist attraction until the explosive ordinance detonation (EOD) team comes to dispose of it. Interpreters arrive to hear their demands and persuade the crowd to disband peacefully. After a few hours, the masses disperse, and the show is over without bloodshed. It is a tense situation, but also an oddly welcomed distraction.

The day started with such high tensions, I suspect it's not yet over. As the early afternoon arrives, I sit on the side of the road, resting my back against the cement pylons of the overpass to ease the weight of my flak. It is quiet, but the scent of war is all around, as is a feeling that the city of Fallujah is restless, like a bubble begging to burst. I continue listening to the radio throughout the day, keeping abreast of operational updates. An order is passed that only women and children will be allowed to leave the city beginning in the afternoon. No cars can enter or leave unless they are carrying medical supplies or food and water. Another order is sent over the radio that anyone wearing black pajamas with a green headband will be arrested or engaged on site.

This is in response to a threat made by a terrorist named Muqtada al-Sadr and his militia called the Mahdi Army, an extremist Shia group pouring out of Baghdad towards Fallujah to "kill Americans." They have adopted this outfit as their clothing of choice for their mission.

It's 1:30 p.m. as I sit on the back bumper of the ambulance picking through my teriyaki chicken MRE. I dash the mini tabasco included in the package to help the bland flavor. A few men play scrabble next to me, others nap on stretchers off to the side of the road in the gravel. My cumbersome flak jacket restricts movement of my chest as I chew, and I feel especially miserable while I eat. It feels hotter than yesterday, but it's likely the same one hundred and something oppressive temperature it has been every other day. I look over at a flytrap we placed on the ground in front of the ambulance, and although it brims with dead flies, they still seem to be abundant in swarms and torment me at every moment. I eat all the chicken and move on to some peanut butter squeezed onto pound cake when I hear the radio buzz. Petty Officer Aircroth answers the call, saying, "This is Med-Man One, send it."

The radio pauses and then squawks back, "Be advised, Med-Man, we are inbound with one severely wounded Marine." We are up and moving before Aircroth puts down the receiver.

As we prepare to receive our injured Marine, another Humvee streams into the cloverleaf unannounced with three wounded insurgents detained in the back of the truck. They are being transported to a detention facility, but before entry require inspection of their injuries. I anticipated this event and hate the responsibility I am charged with—to medically care for these men—plainly speaking, I don't want to care for them. It is difficult for me to contain my resentment. This is war, and they are killing my marines. I look at them staring my way in the back of the Humvee, reminding myself my job is to be a doctor and naval officer—Marines first, all else comes second.

The three insurgents are in handcuffs, lying face-up on our stretchers. As I approach, I smell an awful stench coming from their bodies; it's obvious they have not bathed in weeks.

Their clothing is filthy and tattered. They are all young Arab men who appear to be in their twenties. They are thin framed, with dark features and scant facial hair. I put on gloves and a mask so I can get closer to make a general survey of their wounds. My job is to make sure they are stable for transport to the detention facility. They are cooperative and silent as I look them over with marines standing close by. Their condition ranges from minor cuts and abrasions to gunshot wounds. None of these injuries are life threatening, but one man has an open wound festering on his knee that is badly infected. As I come closer, I am shocked to see maggots squirming in the necrotic pus-filled tissue. What baffles me even more is that he doesn't seem to care.

I would like to tell you I cleaned out the wound of this afflicted soul, but in good conscience, I cannot tell you I did. I let him lie there with his hands securely bound.

I give them water, and my corpsmen stand over them swatting the flies swarming about their faces. Fortunately, their presence is a brief distraction, and they exit shortly in an armed convoy.

Five minutes pass and another Humvee storms into the aid station with our wounded marine who had been called in over the radio. They pull him from the back of the Humvee and instantly I recognize his face; it's Private Erikson! I gasp as I see the extent of his wounds, and then I move towards him. As we transfer him onto the stretcher, our eyes meet, and I know he understands the gravity of his situation. His sergeant approaches, explaining that his platoon was engaged in heavy fire in Fallujah when Private Erikson was directly hit by an RPG. Inexplicably, it did not explode upon impact with his body; rather, it deflected off his left forearm and shoulder, then detonated against the building behind him. The impact of the RPG caused an open fracture of his left forearm and carved a canoe-like path through his deltoid shoulder muscle. It's the largest open wound in a living person who is not in surgery that I have ever seen. Tendons, skin, and muscle hang loosely from where they were once attached. A huge flap of skin and muscle flops to one side, as if it has been carved from his shoulder. The top of his humerus bone is plainly exposed, shiny and white. Uninjured vessels hide sheepishly nearby.

Beyond explanation, he is alive and talking to me as if he just got the wind knocked out of him. Even more remarkable, bleeding is tame, with no major vessels severed. This is partially due to the massive deltoid muscles surrounding his shoulder and otherwise divine intervention.

We put him on a stretcher, and the first thing he says to me is, "Hey, doc, guess we don't need to worry about my forearms anymore."

"Yeah, I think we need to concentrate on your shoulder," I reply.

"I'm sorry, sir, I didn't mean to call you doc," he says, remembering only corpsmen are called "doc," and I am to be called "Doctor."

I reply, "Private, right now you can call me whatever you want. You just take it easy, let us fix you up and get you out of here as soon as possible."

He smiles with a grimace of pain and says, "Thank you, sir, can I have a cigarette?"

I smile back with my hand on his leg and say, "I'll find one for you, Private."

I know he is in shock, probably picturing himself on the cover of *Soldier of Fortune* magazine, toking on a smoke. I don't blame him.

As he smokes, I see the distress on his face as the adrenaline wears off and pain sets in. I give him a morphine injection in the left thigh and then go to work on his shoulder, carefully irrigating his wounds while my corpsmen splint his forearm. I gently replace the large flap of skin and muscle over the wound, to protect exposed vessels and nerves. He has a good pulse and can move his fingers, but I worry about the extent of his injuries. His eyes soften and breathing calms as the morphine sedation sets in. Standing on the side of the road, I keep one eye on him as I look in the distance for the approaching medevac convoy. Another ten minutes pass, though it feels like thirty, and finally, a convoy from Regiment arrives to take him back to the surgical company.

I lean in close before they load him into the Humvee saying, "Hey, war fighter, you will get through this. Stay alert. You're going back to base now, and they will take care of you."

His reply is slow as he turns his eyes towards mine and says in a low tone, "I'll see you soon, sir." He smiles briefly, then it leaves his face. The Humvee engines fire to life and the convoy departs the cloverleaf.

I don't see Private Erikson for five months until we are back in the states at Camp Pendleton, and I'm taken aback when we meet. I am walking into the gym near battalion headquarters when someone calls my name before I reach the door, "Doctor Wilkes, sir!"

I turn to my right and standing on the grass is Private Erikson. I am shocked at the sight of the Marine I once knew; he has lost forty pounds, his entire left arm is atrophied, dwindled to a stick and held at his side. I approach him quickly with my hand held out in earnest, saying, "Private, it's great to see you. How are you doing?"

He doesn't hesitate to reply, "I'm doing okay, but I've lost count of how many surgeries I've had and it's not over."

"My gosh, I can't imagine how rough that has been," I say.

He pauses, and in a more serious tone he says, "Sir, I have to tell you I've been drinking and getting into some trouble. I can't use my arm or do any of the things I used to do. I feel useless."

I pause to digest the weight of his situation. He is reaching out to me, someone who was there at the turn of events in his life. I want to convince him he has everything to live for, to tell him that he's good enough, that he can overcome his injuries and find a new path in life. But I know the daunting uphill battle he has ahead, and I'm worried my words will be inadequate.

I take a deep breath and reply, "Listen, I can't imagine what you have been through since your injury in Iraq. Anyone would struggle after a life-changing event like that, but you can't let this get the best of you; you can't let it define your life. Private, you are one of the best marines I've known, and you have your whole life ahead of you."

He cuts in, "I know it, sir, I just can't seem to control my emotions lately and feel out of control and…"

"There are good people who want to help you," I interject. "I want to help you, and my office is around the corner." I point across the parking lot in the direction of my office.

He pauses thoughtfully, considering my words, and politely says, "Thank you, sir, I understand. I'm trying to take it day by day—doing the best I can."

I don't want to push him too hard; I feel the weight of his struggle. "I know you're trying, Private, and I don't want you to stop. Get the help you need and come find me if you run into problems."

"I will. Thank you, sir." He reaches out, I grab his hand with my right, then my left, we shake, then release, and he walks away. I feel worried about his future, remembering how he liked to live on the edge. I'm hoping this doesn't push him over it. This is the last time I will see or hear anything about Private Erikson.

After Private Erikson leaves the cloverleaf, it is quiet for the rest of the afternoon. Dusk is approaching, usually followed by relief as the heat eases its grip on the city, fighting in Fallujah calms, and our bodies and minds follow suit. I stand in front of the ambulance as I often do to enjoy some shade. Flies buzz about my head; I swat at them without consequence. A few men sit behind me in the gravel embankment, discussing the latest news from headquarters. Despite the intense combat over the last few days, I hear our forces are making progress, advancing farther into Fallujah. We don't know how long we will be at our current position; operational plans change daily. Three corpsmen stand to my left talking and smoking cigarettes. Dirt and gravel shift beneath their feet as they adjust their heavy vests on their backs. Nothing of importance is happening; we are passing time.

In the next moment, before sound can justify the cause, I find myself unsteady on my feet and momentarily deaf from a massive blast. As I try to grasp what happened, the smell of gunpowder hits my nose and my vision is temporarily stunned. I can see people running for cover, so I follow them towards the rear of an open ambulance. *BOOM!* Another concussive round pummels the ground, knocking us unsteady as we run. It's a rocket attack, right on the money. As I stagger to regain my footing, I see the back of the ambulance is almost in reach; Lieutenant O'Connor dives in headfirst and I dive in on top of him, followed by three other Corpsmen behind me. White smoke drifts underneath the overpass as we regain our composure. I breathe heavily, lying face down in the ambulance, dazed and still sorting out what just happened. Other men lie to my right and left; we stay piled together like a rugby team until the explosions stop.

"Is everyone okay?" Lieutenant O'Connor yells from beneath me.

"Yeah, Okay!"

"I'm good, me too!"

"I'm all right." Each of us chimes out, reassuring the pile of men.

"Okay, let's check outside for injuries," Lieutenant O'Connor directs from below. We peel ourselves out of the ambulance one by one. Other men outside are performing the same ritual, rising from the ground, dusting themselves off, and clearing their heads. No one is physically injured, but the emotional damage is fierce.

The rocket attack is shockingly close, a direct hit on our position pounding the western dirt embankment of the cloverleaf. Enemy forces have our position dialed in, and there is nothing we can do about it. U.S. forces follow Geneva convention protocols, defining the basic rights of wartime prisoners, civilians, and protections for the wounded and medical personnel. Our enemy could care less that we are non-combatants providing only medical care; the rules of war are meaningless to them. Marines patrol the perimeter constantly, responding to each attack with counter artillery, but it does not deter the insurgents from sending mortars and rockets right back at us. They cannot be stopped.

Lying awake in the back of my ambulance that night, I am not sad or lonely, but seething over what I cannot do: fight back. It's a helpless feeling, taking me to dark places I have not been before. It's the battle

I don't know how to win, the battle against my own will, to somehow control my situation. My mission is to heal, to sustain life, but death and destruction are dominant and overwhelming. I want to make a deal with God, to make it all go away in exchange for my devotion and commitment to His word, but I know it doesn't work that way.

I'm stuck at the cloverleaf, like or not, and I need to deal with it. Placing my head in my hands, I roll over on the stretcher, pushing the thoughts away and trying to calm the storm.

CHAPTER 11

The Cloverleaf, Day Four, April 11th, 2004 (+117)

Marines in Fallujah use the cloverleaf as a staging ground for many elements of the assault. From the cloverleaf, I watch attack helicopters dive onto their targets like eagles, tanks rumble past like locomotives, and convoys of infantry men storm into the city. Army units join with ours, meeting under the overpass to plan and coordinate attacks. British and Aussie special forces join with our special forces teams to carry out surgical strikes on high-value targets.

Reporters come and go as they follow the Marines and the swings of the battle. Political figures, including the mayor of Fallujah, travel through as they venture into the city, struggling to regain control from the sheikhs. Military supply trains rumble through at all hours of the day or night, dropping off supplies ranging from food and water to ammunition and weapons. They transport new personnel to and from the front lines and occasionally evacuate the wounded. Iraqi ambulances and supply trucks pass through on their way into the city, providing the civilians with medical care, food, and water. Tanks and amphibious assault vehicles convene and stage their positions at the cloverleaf before going out on missions. Heavy gun trucks and marines now occupy all four corners of the cloverleaf, controlling all access to vehicles requesting passage through.

Throughout the night, our marines exchange heavy gunfire and artillery rounds with insurgent forces while I lie in my ambulance, eyes wide open. At 5:30 a.m., I roll off my rack and grab my uniform hanging on the stretcher above me; it is the same uniform I have worn the last four days, now crusty with sweat stains lining the collar. Perhaps tomorrow I will break out the fresh uniform I have tucked away in my pack like a prize. For now, I reunite with the stench of my old one, pulling the legs up over my dirty feet. I strap on my boots and poke my head through the doors.

I smell that someone across the highway has made instant coffee; this is enough to lift my spirits and I join the men.

Throughout the morning, gunfire and bombs echo in the northern section of the city. A third battalion is pushing in from the north, to meet up with our boys coming from the south and the east. The goal is to meet somewhere in the middle of Fallujah, then push west together towards the Euphrates River to solidify control of the entire city.

As the sun drags across the sky into the afternoon, I'm feeling positive; we haven't received any casualties today and intel says our troops are closing in on central Fallujah. First Sergeant Blumenberg is brought to the BAS with a shrapnel wound to his neck. He has made several trips to the cloverleaf in the last few days with both minor and severely injured Marines.

Yesterday I jokingly said to him, "First Sergeant, I don't want to see your face around here anymore unless it's for a good reason!"

He smiled and replied, "I don't want to see you anymore either, sir."

This time, it's he who has a close call. While patrolling the streets, an RPG whizzes past him, exploding on a wall behind him. Fortunately, his wounds are only in the part of his neck that was not covered by his armor. He is lying flat on the stretcher as I approach to survey his face and neck. He has a small piece of shrapnel penetrating the right side, though it's superficial and the bleeding has already stopped.

He tells me, "There is no way I'm being evacuated to the surgical company, so you better remove this shrapnel, doc."

I reply, "I'll do my best, First Sergeant, but if this shrapnel penetrates deeper in your neck, you've won a ticket to the Fallujah day spa back at base."

Reluctantly, he smirks and nods, understanding.

I inspect the wound and see a small piece of shrapnel buried close to the surface. Gingerly, I remove it, then open the wound with a probe to look for any other retained fragments. The wound is clear; I irrigate it and stitch it up with nylon suture. I apply a gauze dressing and give him a five-day supply of antibiotics and pain medication.

"Have your corpsman remove the stitches in five days, First Sergeant," I tell him.

He thanks me, and we exchange a handshake.

"And keep it clean!" I yell as he hustles into the Humvee, peeling off the highway back to the front lines.

As First Sergeant Blumenberg's Humvee fades from sight, a red crescent Iraqi ambulance approaches into the overpass, stopping across the highway from the aid station. The dented white sliding door opens and a frantic Iraqi man wearing black pants and a white short-sleeve shirt steps out and runs directly towards us across the

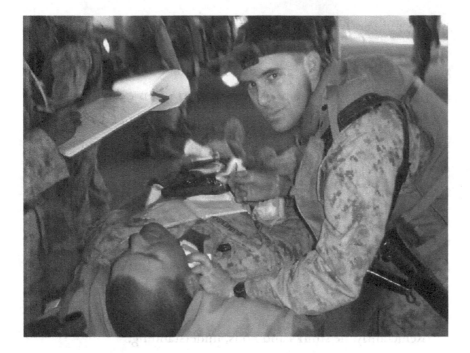

pavement. He is yelling in Arabic and moving erratically; instantly my corpsmen move towards him with raised weapons. As he moves closer, it's obvious his frantic behavior is due to a major facial wound and he's pleading for help. The ambulance driver runs up to assist, grabs him by the arm, and leads him to me.

The Iraqi man continues to scream hysterically. With one look, I see he has a huge flap of skin severed from his face, now hanging off his cheek. There is little time for discussion; my decision-making is brief. With this type of injury, the primary concern is his airway. Since he is talking and yelling at me, I know his breathing is safe for the moment. We are not authorized to take care of Iraqi civilians unless they are brought to us by our military personnel or wounded in combat. I instruct the ambulance driver to take him to the Jordanian hospital just a few miles down the road. As the yelling and pleading persist, he coaxes the Iraqi man back into the ambulance and they speed away. The red crescent ambulances were given access to Fallujah a few days after the battle began, to transport wounded civilians and insurgents to Iraqi hospitals, and we have seen them frequently since. Unfortunately, the ambulances often smuggle weapons to the insurgents, making it difficult to distinguish friend from foe.

My third patient of the day is a young lance corporal suffering from combat stress. His platoon commander brings him to me after he refuses to engage the enemy in Fallujah. It's late in the day, the afternoon sun is begging to retire, yet beads of sweat cling to my brow as I approach him standing in the gravel.

"Take a seat here, Lance Corporal Harrington," I instruct, pointing to the roadside. "I know it must be crazy out there, I hear the fighting from here. I can only imagine how it is on the front lines. Tell me what's going on," I implore.

"Sir, when the enemy starts firing at us...I-I just freeze up," he explains.

"What do you mean by freeze up? What happens?"

He takes and a deep breath before he speaks, and I see it's a struggle for him to recount the events.

"Sir, I am the driver of our Humvee. Today my platoon was taking gunfire and RPGs from across the street. I was ordered to drive our Humvee towards our men to provide fire support, but I couldn't do it. I just froze and couldn't drive forward."

"What do you think is holding you back?" I ask.

"The stress, sir," he states.

"The stress of what?" I probe further.

He hesitates for a moment, and then says firmly, "Dying, sir."

I pause to consider what he said. Then I ask him, "Do you have recurrent thoughts about this?"

His forehead wrinkles, he holds his hands to the side of his head, then he says, "Yes, sir, I have constant images of my friends getting killed, and I dream about it at night."

Harrington was in Iraq one year ago, also in combat situations, and since I joined the battalion he performed well, without hesitation. I need to press him for more details.

"I know you were here last year and did a great job, so what do you think is different this time? What's setting you off?" I ask.

He sighs, then replies, "I don't know; I just saw a couple of my friends get shot two days ago, and ever since then, I can't get my head straight. I feel vulnerable in this fight, much more than the initial invasion of Iraq last year. Back then, we just rolled through with tanks and heavy artillery, blowing everything to hell, but this time our hands are tied, we even have civilians to worry about."

This is a common response I've heard from marines. Despite specific orders to "kill or capture insurgents," they are frustrated about the complexity of fighting an enemy that often disguises themselves as civilians and ignores the rules of modern warfare. Our marines want the gloves off their hands, just like the insurgents. "How are you eating and sleeping?" I ask.

"Not well, sir," he quickly says. His shoulders slump, his head hangs low, he appears dejected. He isn't going to do well if I send him back out.

"Okay, war-fighter, it sounds like you're having some combat stress, and it's not uncommon out here. I don't like taking you out of the fight, but your commander needs you one hundred percent out there. There is no shame in this; the best thing you did is tell us.

What we need to do is send you back to the regimental headquarters to the rest and relaxation center where you can get some hot chow and clear your head for forty-eight hours. Then we'll get you back to the front lines. Sound like a plan?" Having been trained to recognize combat stress, I'm allowed to make this call on the spot. The commanding officer is notified and may overturn my decision, but it's unlikely. They want clear-headed marines on the front lines just as much as I do.

The tension in his brow relaxes. "Yes, sir. Thank you," he replies with an air of relief. "Are you hungry?" I ask.

"Yes, sir," he replies.

I motion for a corpsman to get him food. He sits on the stretcher, quietly eating his food, his head bent, eyes down. When he finishes eating, he wordlessly lies down behind a cement column and sleeps for the next four hours straight without moving a limb.

Evening approaches, and we sit on the ground at the side of the highway, eating MREs and discussing the day's events. The sun is setting on the city; a sherbet-orange haze blankets the skyline above Fallujah and softens the mood. The streets are quiet, and it feels like fighting is over for the day. I scrape the last few bites of my meal from the bottom of the pouch with a long plastic spoon, then throw it in a trash box. Heavy with protein and preservatives, the meal will take a couple of hours to settle.

"Want to play some cards?" Petty Officer Guzman asks. "Sure; why not; what's your game?" I reply.

I stand up and take two steps towards the front of our ambulance. From above, a searing *HISSSS* pierces the sky, escalating like an electric charge. Before my head turns up towards the ungodly sound, a mind-numbing explosion obliterates the western off-ramp of the cloverleaf. Like a rag doll, I hit the ground effortlessly. Temporarily paralyzed, stunned and breathless, I struggle for clarity. The blast is powerful, sending a stampede of shock waves through the overpass, briefly forcing the breath from my lungs. Pissed off, cussing, and confused, I lie on the ground, then slowly pick up my eyes to look around. A gruesome sense of fury lingers in the air; the smell of gunpowder and sulfur circles overhead, and hateful anger fills my brain. I silently scream as I lower my head into my hands. I've never felt this powerlessness before. I feel as if I've lost control over my own life, even my death. I'm here to help others, but my mortality consumes me while another man out in the desert wreaks havoc on me and my men. I want to crush him with my hands, but I can't. There is no one to grab onto, nothing to crush. I know I can lean on Christ; I know He is the spiritual warrior who will see me through, but my training is weak, and I'm not as prepared as I thought. *"I will get back on top,"* I think, *"I will learn how to win."* But at the moment, I am shell-shocked. So, I do what all warriors do. I get up, dust myself off, grit my teeth, and keep moving. I walk through the cloverleaf, check on my men, and prepare the aid station. No one is injured, but the blast has taken its toll.

CHAPTER 12

The Cloverleaf, Day Five, April 12th, 2004 (+ 118)

My path from the tranquil courtyards of New Orleans' French Quarter to the war wounded streets of Fallujah has been a symphony of twists and turns. I feel like I've been running towards and colliding with unknowns, stacking on each other like a staircase to an undiscovered door. As I think about the path, I realize how interconnected both worlds have been to me.

My six years in New Orleans, joining the Navy, navigating a marriage during war, and treating combat casualties have sequenced my life like a beaded necklace. Each step unveiled new obstacles and new thrills that pushed me to seek the next layer of my life. The pursuit of a medical degree gave me confidence to compete at the highest level of intellect. I was an underdog—but like Rocky Balboa, I went fifteen rounds, and I hung with the best. The mystique of life in New Orleans added fuel to the fire—I arrived knowing no one, jumped in headfirst, and put my heart on the line. I sought an adventurous course, and it sought me right back. Joining the Navy solidified that path. Despite the uncertainty and adversity, I learned to trust my instincts, believing the leaps of faith are not as perilous as they may have looked, and my choices were more calculated than they felt. Katie and I put it all on the line choosing a wartime marriage. Her faith in me is the glue that binds, solidifying the courage I needed to depart for war with a full heart and at peace with my fate.

Now I find myself at the unknown pinnacle of my life in Fallujah. I'm entering dimensions I could not have imagined. Men are coming to me in the greatest fight of their life, some persevering in glorious fashion as they fight to serve their country, while others succumb to the ultimate defeat. These events transpire in minutes, as lives are changed in an instant, and these men are lost to me forever.

Despite the contrast of my vibrant life in New Orleans to the dark side of Fallujah, I'm connecting my life's events in a new light. I'm seeing how God's grace has permeated my journey at each crossroad, pushing me into new realms with a loving strength. With each "leap of faith" I'm finding that I'm listening to His call, and it keeps me coming back for more. I'm running towards the light, not the light of flickering gas lamps along St. Charles Avenue, but the light of the Lord, reassuring me that once again, despite the great unknowns ahead, I'm right where I am meant to be.

I'm counting the days, and today is day number five at the cloverleaf. The morning starts like all others: roll out of my rack in the ambulance, electric shave, quick breakfast, situation report, then a routine drama ensues. Machine gunfire in Fallujah pierces the morning calm, an explosion follows shortly after—likely an RPG or grenade. The corpsmen and I are poised in position at the BAS, waiting for a status report. Without radio contact, a Humvee exiting Fallujah comes screaming towards the cloverleaf; plumes of dust spew chaotically in its wake. I stand still and watch it approach from the edge of the highway; this is a familiar and paralyzing dance I have come to know.

My radial pulse trips to a gallop as the urgency builds. It's unmistakable and all but obvious even before face or flesh is seen that this vehicle carries a wounded man. I am on my toes and moving towards them as the tires skid to a halt. Three marines rush from the back carrying the limp body of a wounded marine. His left arm dangles over the side of the stretcher and his head flops to one side. Blood is abundant; multiple voices holler out commands. Too many people are screaming for me to make sense of anything. I spot the company first sergeant among his men. Walking right up to him, I bring him close, my flak jacket to his and I say, loudly, "First Sergeant, tell me what happened!"

The first sergeant still has his helmet on and is sweating profusely, with his M16 in one hand and deep concern on his face. He replies loudly, "Sir, we were heading up a stairwell on a house raid looking for insurgents when we came under sniper fire; Sergeant Boudreaux was shot in the leg, and Corporal Sanders took a round to the head. We returned heavy gunfire while our Corpsmen did all they could at the scene, sir, then we rushed them to you."

"Thanks, first Sergeant, we're going to do everything we can," I say quickly as I move away.

I turn my attention to the treatment area, where men swarm like bees around our marine.

Determined to have everyone's attention, I yell, "Anyone who is not a corpsman needs to get out of the way!"

Fellow marines shout final words of encouragement, then bodies part as my corpsmen and I move in and go to work. My mind is soupy, a bit sluggish, and I take a moment to gather my thoughts.

"Okay, I have been here before. Prioritize: start with the airway and breathing, and the rest will fall into place." Then, I am ready to go.

To my right is Sergeant Boudreaux, shot in the leg. His cammies are cut off, exposing a small circular bullet hole in his right upper thigh. There is localized swelling and minor bleeding from the frayed tissue at the entrance site, but otherwise, he looks stable. I turn his care over to my corpsmen to concentrate on Corporal Sanders, who has sustained a gunshot wound to the head. I heave a deep breath, feeling my chest strain against my flak, then twist my body to the left, take a few steps forward, and place myself at the head of our marine. Commotion surrounds him, sweat and heat radiate from my head. *"Focus, stay calm,"* I remind myself. I look down at the bloody bandages on his head, steady my hand, and peel back one edge to assess the extent of his wounds. I know it's going to be bad, but I am not prepared for what I see; the bullet has entered the left back side of his head and exited through his forehead, leaving a gaping wound; pieces of brain matter cling to skull bones and blood pools in the cavernous wound. All I can think is, *"My dear God, how is this man still alive?"*

I am painfully aware that no matter what we do to save his life, his chances of survival are extremely slim, and even if he lives, he will have severe brain damage. My thoughts race, things are progressing fast. He has an IV with fluids running, new bandages are placed around his head. I think, *"Should I try to prolong his life or let things end here?"*

We discussed these scenarios during field medical training, but nothing could have prepared me for this moment. I glance up, looking beyond our stretcher. Marines cling to their weapons and stand shoulder to shoulder, staring earnestly at their fallen brother. I look back at his face; he is still breathing on his own, moving his eyes but otherwise unresponsive. I rub my fist on his sternum, looking for a response to pain, but he is motionless. My decision takes mere seconds and the choice becomes clear; we will proceed with all-out efforts, because our marines looking on should see nothing less.

Initially, I place a curved plastic mouthpiece into his oral cavity to keep his tongue from falling to the back of his mouth, obstructing his airway. I turn to a corpsman and say, "Put a face mask over his nose and mouth and turn the oxygen up to fifteen liters per minute."

Another corpsman quickly irrigates and packs the large exit wound on his forehead with gauze to minimize bleeding. Fluids are running in his IV, and I ask for one gram of Ancef antibiotic to be given. I decide I will not give him morphine because his blood pressure and respirations are tenuous and this could depress them further.

A few minutes tick by as we complete these tasks, and I notice his breathing is labored and he is beginning to cough up blood. His upper body gently kicks with each spatter of blood flying from his mouth. Tensions rise as I hover over his head, attempting to sort it out in my brain and with my hands. I remove the oral airway and decide to attempt an endotracheal intubation to help him breathe. For this procedure, I use a laryngoscope, an instrument with a long dull metal blade and a light source to view his vocal cords, to advance a breathing tube into his trachea.

As I prepare for the procedure, I try to pry open his mouth with my fingers to look at his throat, but his teeth are clenched tight. "Now what?" I mumble under my breath. I cannot place the laryngoscope into his mouth to perform the intubation, and I don't have the medications I need to paralyze his jaw muscles so he will not clench his teeth.

Things get worse; he starts bucking and spitting up more blood, causing him to choke. Two men hold him down, blood spatters on my face and onto his chest. "*Oh God, I don't want anyone to see it end this way,*" I think. We turn his head to the side, then use a suction tube to clear blood from the back of his throat. This stops his choking for the moment, but I fear the bleeding from his head wound will continue to drain down his throat into his lungs—I need to secure a reliable airway. The ground medevac is inbound; we must work fast before he is loaded on a Humvee. Seconds tick by; anguish and fervor fill my heart. I decide to place a surgical airway.

I yell to my corpsman, "I need a cric kit!" (That's a cricothyrotomy kit, used to make an incision to establish an airway.)

Usually, there is one right next to me, but as I glance to my left and right, and left again, it's not there; my nerves mount. Behind me, scrambling among boxes and equipment, my corpsmen look frantically for the kit. Corporal Sanders continues to choke and spit up blood, again I repeat my request, now with desperation, "I need that cric kit now!"

The search intensifies, but still no luck. Boots shuffle louder and faster in the dirt around the stretcher. His head bobs up as he chokes, and again I suction his airway to clear the blood. Just when I am about to improvise a different method for the procedure, my corpsman hands me the cric kit. Quickly, I begin. I ease a long, large needle from the kit at forty-five degrees through the skin just below his Adam's apple, then through subcutaneous fat and tissue, and finally through a thin membranous window allowing entrance into the sacred airway. My thumb and index finger grip the needle firmly. "*Hold it steady; don't lose it,*" I think. Next, I place a thin plastic dilator into the lumen of the needle and the airway, allowing me to safely break away the rigid plastic needle.

"Okay, hold the dilator," I tell my corpsman; his hand replaces mine.

I reach into the instrument tray, grab a small blade, and make a vertical incision to widen the entrance into his airway, allowing the dilator to slide further inside. He still struggles to breathe as we work, panting blood and air. Success is near; *"Just a minute more,"* I think. I slide the curved plastic airway tube over the dilator and halfway into his trachea before encountering resistance. I push harder—once, twice, but still can't advance all the way. I make the incision larger, then try again. *"Yes, we're home,"* I tell myself, breathing a heavy sigh of relief as the tube slides snugly into his airway. Finally, I inflate a small plastic bag-like cuff on the end of the tube to seal the airway, keeping blood from draining into his lungs.

"Suction the tube every five minutes to keep it open," I instruct my corpsman. Almost instantly, breathing eases and he stops choking. I step back, inspecting the stability of his airway. The crisis is over for the moment, and corpsmen join me with brief glances of success to each other.

His airway is secure, the bleeding from his head wound has tapered; I survey the rest of his body for other wounds. He has bruising and swelling over his right upper chest, and his breath sounds are diminished on the right side of his lungs. I'm confused about how he sustained trauma to this region and concerned it may be secondary to blunt force or a blast injury causing air trapping around his lungs. If progressive, air trapping can accumulate, leading to respiratory failure if not released. I decide to place a large needle into his upper lung space to see if this improves his breathing. I locate a safe entrance point between his second and third ribs on his right upper chest. I advance the needle almost three inches into his chest, hoping to hear a rush of air release, but there is none. I listen to his lungs again. The air is moving freely with an equal expansion of both sides; however, he remains unconscious, only breathing ten times per minute. He is breathing on his own, but he is still in critical condition. I pray the ambulance will arrive shortly as there is nothing else I can do. His fellow marines and sailors look on with angst.

The ambulance pulls into the overpass a few minutes later. Sergeant Boudreaux and Corporal Sanders are loaded onboard. One of my senior corpsmen jumps on board to continue suctioning the airway tube. We close the back doors; they speed away among a procession of Humvees and seven-ton trucks mounted with heavy machine guns. All we can do is pray.

Thirty minutes later we receive word over the radio that he is in surgery, still in critical condition. I cannot help wondering if God should take him into His loving arms now; if he survives the odds of any semblance of a normal life are next to none, but I know these uncertainties are not for me to decide. A short time later we learn he died shortly after surgery during transport to another hospital. Another life is lost, and our hearts are heavy. I walk among the men, to thank them and be with them.

"You all performed bravely today. I'm proud of you." I say.

For some of them, it's the first time they have seen a wounded man die.

"Do you think the surgical airway worked?" inquires Petty Officer Martinez.

"Yes, it got him to the surgical team, so it was the best we could do," I reassure him. "I know it's bittersweet today, but you performed well, prolonging a life that ended in defeat, and there is no shame in that," I say sincerely.

"I hope that's all for today, sir," he says with a tired sigh.

"Me too, Martinez, me too," I say.

"It's going to be dark soon, let's get this mess cleaned up and grab some food," I insist.

"Yes, sir, I'll grab some MREs," he replies and shuffles away to the pile of food boxes next to our medical supplies. He rifles through the box as if the best one might magically appear. Another corpsman goes to the front of the ambulance, grabs the radio receiver, and notifies command headquarters Corporal Sanders has died. MREs are handed out, and as we each take a seat around the back of the ambulance, the conversation is minimal. After dinner, the sun is setting at the aid station; a few corpsmen light cigarettes, gathering in a small circle. They stand in the advancing shadows, a few feet from me, puffing slowly and talking. I see the embers waft gently to the ground, like incendiary snowflakes. A gentle breeze shifts and the tobacco plumes reach my nose. I don't smoke, but the smell is good, and I want to be with the men.

Without getting up I say, "Hey, Martinez, how about you give me one of those smokes?"

He turns my way with a surprising look and says, "I didn't know you smoked, sir."

"I don't, but I will tonight," I respond, smiling.

He smiles back, reaching for his pocket. I get up, he meets me halfway with a cigarette extended in his hand, then provides a light and I join the circle of men. With one eye, my corpsmen look at me curiously as we stand together, lingering in the light of dusk. I catch glimpses of their faces and I know they understand; the smoking is a gesture we are in this fight together. The sun is yellow-orange meringue, softened as it gently sets over the war-torn city. From the islands of the Pacific during WWII, to the jungles in Vietnam, I know our circle is a replica of those that have transpired during war for decades—and I like it. I listen to them talk, finding peace in their conversation and comfort remembering our common mission, why we're here: to support our warriors, the marines and sailors now dug into the hollows of Fallujah. They will not give up, and we won't leave until we all go together.

It's been a tragic day, bullish and unpredictable. Now more than ever I understand death has no consideration of my preparedness and is boldly indifferent to my fears. More than expected, it has become larger than life. These are the challenges at the cloverleaf, and I am keenly aware that time is not my friend. When each day begins, I am ready for it to end; the more I fight it, the more it fights back. I'm learning to rely on God's grace, to lean on His strength as it calls to me time and time again, yet I am afflicted, and sometimes distracted. Still I feel God's presence, and I know He is with me, seeking my friendship with an outstretched hand. My hand is reaching too; I'm getting close, and I know He will never give up on me.

TIME OFF THE LINE

Almost a week after coalition forces unilaterally suspend offensive military operations in Fallujah, the overall situation in and around the city remains unchanged. Provocative attacks continue in Fallujah despite the ceasefire, and anti-coalition forces in Fallujah continue to use local mosques for weapons storage. The insurgents continue to fortify their positions by building roadblocks in the city and stockpiling weapons. Fighters have ransacked numerous homes, taking them over and forcing residents out.

I have been at the cloverleaf since April 8th, and it's time for me to transfer back to Camp Mercury. I raise Cormac on the radio in the morning to make arrangements for our switch. "Medicine Man Two, this is Medicine Man One, over."

Sitting in the cramped passenger side of our ambulance, I hold the black radio receiver in my lap and pause for thirty seconds to allow him time to respond. Moments later the receiver squawks to life. "Medicine Man One, send it."

"Cormac, will you be heading to my position today? Over," I reply

"Be advised I will be arriving around 10:00 a.m. this morning on a resupply convoy passing through your position at the cloverleaf. I will relieve you and you can board the convoy back to base. Copy? Over."

"Loud and clear. See you soon. Over and out," I say.

In anticipation, I roll up and cinch my down sleeping bag, fill my daypack with my belongings, and tell my men that I will board the convoy after Lieutenant O'Connor is dropped off to take my place. At 9:45 a.m., I hear the convoy train in the distance; my head tilts up and I can see a Marine in the turret of the leading truck, his hands gripping a fifty-caliber machine gun. Goggles and a neck gaiter obscure his face from thick dust clouds spewing from the tires. The diesel engines echo loudly as the trucks lumber into the overpass, pull up next to our aid station, and come to a halt. The engines purge compressed gas and the steel frames moan to a stop.

I grab my day pack from the back of the ambulance and hurry towards the rear of the trucks, eager to meet my friend and replacement. I see Cormac leap from the back of a Humvee and I hustle towards him, knowing we will only have a few moments to talk. As we shake hands he says, "Hope you're hanging in there."

"It's been quiet so far this morning," I say.

He nods with a smirk, acknowledging this can change at any moment.

"I sent Katie an email to let her know you were unable to call her, but that you're safe.

Can you send the same message to Jen in three days?" He asks.

"Of course; I'll be sure to remember," I say.

I hear the convoy engines growling to life and preparing to move. We shake hands as I say, "Good luck brother, let's talk on the radio within twenty-four hours."

I step away from the shaded overpass into the bright sunshine, walking past our green ambulance on the side of the highway and find an open seat in a Humvee towards the middle of the convoy train. We storm away towards Fallujah. On the way back to Camp Mercury, the convoy needs to resupply Marines posted at fighting positions within the city. As we drive, I see the streets are a graveyard of trash and sewage. Rusted metal, cracked cement, broken glass, and refuse lines almost every path. At predetermined drop spots, we deposit pallets of water, boxes of food, ammunition, and medical supplies. The stops are as brief as possible. Marines dismount each time to establish a guarded perimeter while supplies are offloaded.

Without resistance, we finish the resupply and leave the outskirts of Fallujah. As we bounce along towards Camp Mercury, my head rests against the steel door, rocking gently inside my helmet. The inside of our Humvee smells like dirt, oil, and old clothing, like an old work truck that has seen too many years. I watch passively as we drive through empty terrain, wondering how so much chaos and hate can occupy a single region of the world. My body is tired, and I think about the hot shower awaiting me at the base. I feel like we've had some of the hardest days yet, and I'm hoping the worst is behind us. I tell myself to make it through one day at a time to the next day and the next, until one of those next days becomes the day I go home. My body smells of sweat, and I muse how this blends nicely with everything around me, and that no one is the wiser—not the Humvee driver, not the Marine riding shotgun, or the turret gunner to say the least. We are in this together.

Upon arrival at Camp Mercury, I head straight to my room inside the BAS and unload my gear. I open my day pack and hold it upside down, pouring its contents onto the floor. There are leftover MRE items that I promptly throw away. I have dirty socks and underwear sealed in Ziploc bags and I set them aside for hand washing tomorrow. We have laundry service trucks that haul off weekly loads to another base, but the turnaround time is unpredictable, so I've been doing my laundry old west style, scrubbing my clothes in a bucket on a washboard. After a quick organization of the rest of my gear, I head to the shower trailer. Fortunately, we have hot water today. It's not uncommon to be out, requiring a cold bucket of water for rinsing. Marines and sailors routinely spend a week or more without a shower. After living at the cloverleaf, I've developed a new appreciation for the hardships they endure. Even the port-a-johns are a welcome sight in comparison to a hole in the ground or the dirt-filled boxes we use at the cloverleaf. Turning the knob to full flow, I feel the water splashing in my hair and down my back, bringing a sensation of calm I've not felt for days. I spend a few extra guilty minutes lingering under the hot water, hoping it will not run out for the next person. As I linger, I think about the meal I'll eat tonight. It will likely consist of a meat, perhaps a boiled chicken breast or hamburger served out of a large steaming aluminum bin; a starch like instant mashed potatoes or white rice sprinkled with parsley; and finally, a canned vegetable, usually a green one, like peas, green beans, or both mixed with carrots. The food reminds me of the cafeteria food I ate in middle school and in a strange way the fondness I have for that time in my life. Regardless of the menu, my dinner tonight will be a welcome change from the usual MREs.

After dinner, I call Katie on a satellite phone. Standing outside the BAS, I have to walk around to get a clear signal. It's the longest we have not spoken since starting the deployment. Her voice sounds wonderful, sweet and full of life. As we talk, it's difficult for me to detach myself from the events in recent days. However, I can't tell her any details about events at the cloverleaf. Operational security measures prohibit discussion of any sensitive details that could inadvertently give up information to the wrong people. I can't discuss specifics about our mission, location, or timeline. Nor can I talk about injured marines, sailors, or combatants. Family members of deceased or wounded military personnel must be informed through the proper chain of command, rather than via the rumor mill of deployed marines.

On one hand, I want to pour my heart out to her, to tell her what my eyes have seen and that sometimes I hold my head in my hands at night. But more than this I need to hear about happy things and forget where I am. I want to hear about her simple joys to remind me of the normal life that waits for me. And so she tells me about her new job, and how the weather at the ocean was especially beautiful yesterday. She says the yellow rose bushes are blooming, but the purple hydrangeas are dying. She started painting the kitchen pastel green but had to start over because she didn't like the color, and I laughed when she told me that she bought a Japanese fighting fish to keep her company until I come home. I think about her smile as we talk, and how I've missed her voice. By the time we say goodbye I'm feeling whole again, and I know I can endure. I will do anything to earn the right to go home to her.

After talking with Katie, I decide to watch a movie on my laptop computer in my room. It's been peaceful since arriving at the base. No interruptions from anyone in the BAS or other administrative duties. I look forward to losing myself in a movie for a couple hours. I sit in a metal folding chair with my headphones on; the room is dark and my feet rest on the cold concrete floor in my eight by eight-foot room. I turn up the volume on the movie so I can't hear noise beyond the camouflage blanket hanging over my doorway. For the next two hours, I let the sounds and scenery take me somewhere else, briefly forgetting my place and time as I watch the film.

I wish I could show what happens next, since my words and description may not do it justice. The movie ends and credits parade down the screen as the theme song plays in my headphones. With my right index finger, I reach to press the "enter" button on the keyboard to stop the movie. At the exact instant that my finger depresses the button, a high-pitched hissing sound breaks the sky above me, as if a thousand snakes are descending upon my room. Before I can release my finger and look up towards the ceiling, rockets crush the ground outside, exploding one after another.

My room shakes like an earthquake and the windows rattle violently as I'm thrown to the floor. I'm now face down on all fours, looking about like a wild animal. My ears are ringing and thoughts are fuzzy. Instinctively, I reach out for my helmet on the ground in front of me, scooping it onto my head. I crawl under the blanket in my doorway into the BAS to see if anyone knows what happened. A few corpsmen are just getting to their feet, looking at each other with perfect amazement. We need to check outside for injured marines, but I tell them to hold a minute to be sure the incoming rounds have stopped. The rockets were powerful, enough to take down the toughest of warriors. We sit there staring at each other, stunned and bewildered about what just happened to us.

A few moments later the BAS doors fly open and injured marines with arms around each other stumble into the treatment bay. As corpsmen tend to them, I start moving through the men, scanning faces and bodies for signs of injury. I spot Gunnery Sergeant Johnson with two shrapnel wounds to his head. He is conscious and alert but still in shock as he staggers towards me. I grab his arm and lead him to a chair. He has a stunned look of frustration in his eyes like he just got sucker punched.

"I was in the phone tent, doc, talking to my brother. Next thing I know shrapnel comes ripping through the tent!" he explains.

"I'll take care of you, Sergeant; just relax," I say. He has one piece of metal lodged above his right eye and another near his left temple. A small trickle of bright red blood seeps from both wounds. With a clean metal instrument, I gently probe the puncture site, and I'm relieved to find it's superficial, without penetration to deeper tissue.

The laceration above his eye is stellate-shaped and takes five nylon stitches to close. I wear my helmet and flak jacket while I hunch over and work on him, gladly accepting the discomfort rather than taking the heavy gear off. The sergeant is shaken up; this is his second combat injury since we arrived, and like others, he is wondering if his nine lives are running out.

Next, I turn my attention to another marine. I recognize him as he limps towards me—it's Corporal Menendez. He's thin, about 140 pounds, with dark brown hair and gentle dark brown eyes. I've seen him recently for a gunshot wound to his right leg. He was also in the phone tent when the rocket hit, sustaining shrapnel to his back. It's just a scrape, but this poor fellow is still hobbling around on crutches from his gunshot wound. He asks if I know how he can let his family know he's all right.

"I was on the phone with my wife when the rocket hit," he explains. "We lost connection and I need to tell her I'm okay."

"I'll get you a phone Corporal, no problem," I say. I grab an Iridium satellite phone from the communications shop so he can make his call.

By the time we finish caring for injuries at the BAS, it's nearly 2:00 a.m. I'm exhausted. Too tired to care, I lie down on my mattress and fall asleep, still wearing my uniform and flak jacket.

The next morning, I walk the base to survey the damage. In my room, I was fifty meters from the nearest impact, though I could have sworn it landed on my head. The first rocket hit outside the chow hall next to a seven-ton truck. Twisted hunks of steel surround a gaping hole into the front end and broken glass litters the ground. The driver's side door was blown off, and now the whole truck dips downward from damage to the tire rim and axle, like an elephant kneeling on its front haunches. Another rocket hit near the phone tent, sending shrapnel tearing through the tent walls, inflicting more mental than physical damage to those who were inside. A third rocket made a direct hit on one of the officer tents. Outside the entrance, evidence of our enemy's weapon sticks out of the ground. The casing of a rocket has lodged itself deep in the dirt, and a small crater surrounds the pierced earth. Walking in the tent, I feel as if I'm under a jungle canopy; rays of sunshine and slats of dusty light pierce hundreds of holes in the roof and side walls. My eyes widen when I see the chaos of twisted metal bed frames and shredded personal items strewn everywhere. I can barely make my way from one end of the tent to the other without tripping on the carnage. God's protection was with us last night—all the members of that tent happened to be off base on a mission during the attack. Anyone who slept here surely would have been killed.

CHAPTER 13

The Soda Factory, April 21st, 2004 (+127)

After three days at Camp Mercury, I transport back to the cloverleaf. We're now over two weeks into the attack on Fallujah. I'm sitting in the front passenger seat of the ambulance this morning just staring into space, wondering what the day might have in store, when the radio screeches to life.

"Medicine Man One, Medicine Man One, this is Geronimo, over."

I pick up the receiver and respond, "This is Medicine Man One, send your traffic."

"Medicine Man, be advised you need to pack up your supplies and prepare to move the BAS to the forward COC at the soda factory within one hour. Little Wolf will meet you at the cloverleaf to escort you in," he replies.

I want to know more about the sudden orders to change our position, but I know now is not the time.

"Roger that, we'll be ready to move within one hour. Medicine Man over and out," I reply.

I step out of the ambulance and announce, "We're moving to the soda factory, so pack up the ambulances with all our gear and be ready to head out within an hour."

Part of me is glad to be leaving the cloverleaf, yet another part of me is curious about the implications of why we were leaving. I suspect the order for our move can only mean one of two things. The first is that the enemy is standing down, and we're consolidating our battalion for movement back to Camp Mercury. The other is the insurgents are dug in, requiring us to stage our attacks anew so that the entire battalion can push deeper into the city. In either case, we're on the move, albeit deeper into Fallujah, and for better or for worse it stirs new life into us.

The soda factory is located two miles inside Fallujah. Insurgent forces had taken over this factory by force, using it as an outpost for local raids. As our marines attacked Fallujah, they handily pushed them out, taking it over and establishing the Battalion forward Command Operations Center. The battalion commander resides here and conducts day-to-day operations for the battle in Fallujah.

The soda factory consists of two large hollow buildings, containing all production line equipment for a variety of Iraqi sodas. As I walk into the factory, I'm surprised at how modern it looks. After stashing my gear, I take a walk by myself through the factory. In the main section, the marines set up workspaces. This is where I'm told to establish the new BAS. The remainder of the factory is dark and uninhabited, so I take a flashlight with me to look around. The factory has an aura of unrest; it appears to have been ransacked amid operations. Equipment and tools are abandoned out in the open, unfinished soda products line the assembly tracks, frozen in motion. Large pressure gauges connected to pipes run overhead, many of them eventually leading to a back warehouse with huge steel brewing tanks for the soda. There are large barrels of brown sugar sitting open against the wall. In the corner, I spot some sleeping bags, where a few marines made their beds. Another back room looks like a science lab. There are test tubes, burners, and glass beakers scattered about the room. Most of the glass cabinets have been smashed and broken into.

Throughout the factory, pallets of soda cans are stacked to the ceiling, some full of soda, others are empty aluminum cans without lids. Marines have stacked the pallets of cans to make cave-like shelters to sleep in. The battalion commander purchased the entire stock of soda in the factory from the local owner, allowing us to take as much as we wanted. There are many flavors to choose from, including lemon lime, grape, root beer, and my personal favorite, mandarin orange. This particular brand has real chunks of mandarin orange in the soda; when chilled, it makes a refreshing drink on a hot day. I make my bed in one of the small back offices, placing stacks of cardboard on the ground for a mattress and my down sleeping bag on top. Sacks of crystal sugar are piled high on top of a desk against the windows to protect us from incoming mortars.

Once settled, I head to the COC to find out the status of the battle in Fallujah and the plans for our medical team. The conflict is presently at a standstill, as a ceasefire was called while those in peace talks debated a non-violent ending to the conflict. The U.S.-led coalition had been allowing food, water, and medical supplies into the city since the beginning of the battle, and now they are also allowing some families and vehicles back in as a good-faith gesture.

Before coalition forces will agree to leave Fallujah, insurgents are instructed to halt all attacks and hand over large stockpiles of weapons. It remains to be seen if they will comply with these demands.

Stability in Fallujah is fragile at best. I have little confidence we've seen the end of resistance within the city, and I'm very skeptical to hear we are bargaining with them rather than forcibly completing the occupation of the city. For now, the soda factory is my new home, and I'm content to be living in a structure with four hard walls and a roof over my head and marines at every entrance.

I spend four days at the soda factory while the battle in Fallujah remains at a standstill. The days are slow and uneventful, save for a few mortar attacks around the outer walls of the factory compound. I treat a few marines for minor wounds and illnesses, but no one with serious trauma. The primary struggle each day is to stay busy, fighting the monotony. I think constantly about when I can get the hell out of here.

In front of the factory is a large dirt lot serving as our motor pool. Humvees are parked on one side. On the other is a tin roof awning where broken down vehicles can receive maintenance. The terrain in and around Fallujah wreaked havoc on our vehicles, so repairs were vital to operational readiness. In the back of the motor pool, the marines have constructed a field outhouse.

There are two open stalls with a small piece of plywood between them, just low enough so you will surely feel awkward when someone is sitting next to you. Each "toilet" is made of three cement blocks stacked upwards in a rectangle shape with a hollow center. A hole has been dug in the dirt ground below them. After you do your business, a shovel is handy to throw some more dirt on top. With the temperature usually in the one hundreds daily and endless swarms of flies, I can honestly say this is a humbling and filthy experience.

But I didn't have to build it or maintain it, and there were marines who did, so I dared not complain. Jobs like these were generally delegated to the junior enlisted men, for whom I had the greatest respect. They were the real muscle within the battalion who made everything important happen, from building outhouses, to putting bullets down range.

Beyond the cover of the motor pool, the marines dug foxholes throughout a large open dirt area of the lot. These function as "fighting holes" if marines are engaged in a firefight and serve as protection during rocket and mortar attacks. Beyond the foxholes, a company of tanks is parked against the back wall. They come and go as needed while the battle surges.

In the evening I lie on top of my sleeping bag, on the cases of cardboard soda boxes. It's too hot to sleep under the covers, so I lie on top, staring blankly around my dwelling. All of it is without shadow in the dark; no features can be discerned. The mosquitoes are out in force, so I spray myself each night with copious, sticky repellent that clings to my skin and sleeping bag. An unstable ceiling fan creaks overhead, providing a weak but welcome breeze. I have a care package from home with magazines, food items, and letters. I pull out some chocolate and read a magazine with my flashlight. It has an article about the battle in Fallujah, and as I read, I'm shocked to find key details about the battle are inaccurate and misleading. I know this because I had just lived it and spoke directly with the operations officers who knew all the details of the operation. In essence, the article portrayed the marines as big bullies, attacking the city without regard for its citizens. The article tells blatant lies about how people are treated, and beyond that it's sympathetic towards the insurgents! I can't believe what I'm reading. This isn't some no-name pamphlet, either; it's a major American magazine that millions of people read. That night, I fall asleep frustrated and bitter.

On April 27th, insurgents attack U.S. defensive positions, hindering the ongoing "ceasefire" and forcing coalition forces to call in air support from the George Washington aircraft carrier; laser-guided bombs pummel insurgent positions, pushing them into remission.

Facing growing criticism from the Iraqi Governing Council for civilian casualties, the United States announces withdrawal from Fallujah on May 1st, and we are ordered to regress to Camp Mercury. Lieutenant General James Conway, commanding general of First Marine Expeditionary Forces, states he will turn over any remaining operations to the newly formed Fallujah Brigade, a Sunni-led security force armed with U.S. weapons and equipment under the command of former Ba'ath party member, Major General Mohammed Latif. The hope is that the brigade will maintain stability within Fallujah and limit further bloodshed.

Word spreads fast. Many in our battalion, including myself, are very skeptical about our decision to withdraw from Fallujah before it's secure. However difficult the decision, to the men on the ground it feels like we're giving in to pressure from the Iraqi government and the media, leaving a job half-finished. I understand there have been a lot of civilians displaced and killed from the battle, but I also know leaving prematurely could mean even more death and displacement for them in the future. I'm feeling uneasy about the decision and suspect the mounting political pressure is weighing heavy on our military commanders. Brave marines, sailors, and soldiers have died to gain crucial ground in Fallujah and leaving prematurely could be disastrous.

Sadly, in short order my fears are confirmed; by September of that year, the Fallujah Brigade dissolves and turns over all the U.S. weapons back to the insurgency. The brigade soldiers declare loyalty to the insurgency and other warlords vying for control of the city. Unrest and violence promptly follow, and this eventually ignites the Second Battle of Fallujah in November of 2004. Ultimately, the entire city is occupied by coalition forces but at the cost of many more American and Iraqi lives.

CHAPTER 14

Grace Under Fire, May 17th, 2004 (+153)

It's 1:30 a.m. and I'm asleep in my room when I hear a Corpsman speak up outside my door. "Lieutenant Wilkes, sir! Are you awake? We need you at the BAS," he shouts. I'm half asleep but hear enough to process his request. I shove on my boots, reach for my headlamp, and grab my stethoscope.

"A Humvee was hit by an IED, the initial reports say no serious injuries, but they are bringing the injured marines to the BAS for treatment," he continues.

The cot where I sleep is in a small room inside the BAS, so all I have to do is roll out and take ten steps to be inside our clinic. Eight marines escorted by corpsmen walk into the BAS fifteen minutes later. The dazed look on their faces tells me they are shaken up, but at first glance, I don't notice any serious injuries. They scatter around the room while my corpsmen split up to attend to them, and in an instant our small aid station is alive with commotion and storytelling. Voices peak and trough, arms wave with fervor as accounts of peril and bravery are retold. Some men stand, while others plop themselves on the ground, dropping their dirty packs beside them or stashing their weapons against a wall. Corpsmen buzz around the room taking blood pressures, listening to lung sounds, and dressing wounds. I scan the room from side to side, looking for marines who need the most urgent attention, given away by an ashen face, unsteady gait, or blood on their clothes. They all look and smell like combat action; their clothing is stained with a mixture of sweat, dirt, and grease from their M16s. Small shreds of shrapnel wounds stand out on their light brown desert digital cammies. I inspect each marine briefly, looking for actively bleeding wounds. Three have minor shrapnel wounds that will require only cleaning and dressing. Five others have perforated ear drums from the shockwave of the blast; these do not require emergent treatment but need close follow up to ensure the defect heals. Captain Graham has the most serious injury, a two-centimeter puncture wound in his left hip. Initially, he tells me it's just a bruise and is surprised to find the wound when I cut open his cammies. We wash it out, probe for retained shrapnel, and find none. I leave it open, pack it with gauze, and give him antibiotics for ten days. When Lieutenant O'Connor and I finish treating the injured marines, I ask Chaplain Hall to say a prayer. We huddle together, surrounding the injured men in the BAS while Chaplain Hall prays for healing, protection, and strength.

That night, the blown-up Humvee is towed to our base, and looking at the destruction of the vehicle, I'm amazed no one was more seriously injured. The IED detonated underneath the Humvee, producing a blast wave strong enough to rip through the metal undercarriage and concussive force powerful enough to rupture all their eardrums. IEDs have been a problem for quite some time since the insurgents gained a stronghold in Anbar Province. These homemade bombs are a serious problem because they are cheap, easily constructed, and remotely detonated. Early versions required a wire connection for detonation, but advancements have led to cellular phone devices, removing risk from the missions and emboldening IED campaigns. For the marines, it requires a constant watch for suspicious roadside threats and vigilant patrol of insurgent routes to mitigate new IEDs.

A CORPORAL'S QUEST FOR GRACE

That next Sunday I attend church service with fifteen other marines and sailors at 6:00 p.m. The chapel consists of rows of chairs placed in the back of the chow hall and a folding table for a podium. Lieutenant Wayne Hall is the battalion chaplain. While marines are off base in the field, he conducts site visits, providing support and brief services. Now, since the Battle of Fallujah ended, he provides Sunday service for anyone who can attend. Those who have bibles bring them, and Chaplain Hall has extras for those who don't. He has printed some worship songs from the internet, and we start the service with spirited but generally subpar singing. One of my corpsmen is a large black man I would never guess has a singing voice, but this day he surprises us all with wonderful tenor notes. Our impromptu chapel smells of dust and food left on the floor from lunch; the walls are yellow and smudged with dirt, the windows are cracked with sandbags obscuring the view, but it's the place we gather to honor God, and I feel his presence today. Chaplain Hall preaches for thirty minutes, filling us with strength, hope, and perseverance. We sing and laugh together, briefly forgetting we're in the middle of a vicious and violent part of the world.

On the walk back to the BAS, I hear feet crunching in the gravel as a marine hustles up next to me; it's Lance Corporal Rosales. "Sir, can I ask you a personal question?"

"Sure, go right ahead," I reply.

His dark brown eyes stare up at me. He is five feet, five inches tall with dark brown skin and a dark shaved head. He is lean, weighing only 130 pounds, and his cammies are faded and stained. I remember him from a few nights before; he is one of the marines who survived the IED attack. His oversized M16 bobs gently on his chest as he walks, and after taking a moment to gather his thoughts he asks, "You believe in God, right sir?"

"Yes...I do."

"Well sir, I have been trying to change my ways while I'm out here...I want to be a better person," he says.

"Those are noble and worthy goals."

With a hesitant voice, he responds, "Sir, what I am worried about is that I have almost been killed three times." Lowering his head, we continue down the gravel path, now giving way to dirt and sand.

He continues, "I feel like God is trying to tell me something. Do you think God is sending me a message, sir?"

We slow our strides as we approach the outside walls of the BAS, the faint evening light outlines his silhouette, I can see the whites of his eyes as he looks at me.

I take a moment to consider his question, then say, "I can understand why you might be confused right now, and I'm sure your close calls with death must have been terrible. What is it you think God is trying to tell you?"

He quickly replies, "Sir, like I said, I have been trying to change my ways, but I keep failing, and then bad things keep happening.

I'm trying to do good, but I don't always succeed. I feel like God might be sending me a warning or something. Does God work that way?"

It is nearly dark now as we approach the plywood double doors of the aid station. I ask him to sit with me on a dirt-filled barrier set against the beige stucco wall. I take a deep breath before speaking.

"Rosales, here is the way I look at what happened to you and your question about God's message. First of all, it's clear God is seeking your attention, or we wouldn't be having this conversation. I can't explain the mysterious ways God seeks us, but I can tell you this: I see your close calls with death as small miracles.

"The fact you walked away from that Humvee is unreal, not to mention that you were wounded in combat and involved in another vehicle accident, rolling over four times and coming out almost unharmed! Now, here you are sitting in front of me telling me you want Christ to change your life. Think about how amazing this is by itself. I don't think God wants bad things to happen to you...I think He is telling you He is not done with you yet and He wants to keep you on this earth! It's clear to me God is working through you, making changes to mold you. I can't explain how God responds to each of our imperfections, but I do know this: if you accept God as your savior, believing in his grace, God will forgive you for any wrongs you have done. You can never do enough good deeds to earn God's forgiveness, but Jesus earned it for you when He died on the cross, so all you have to do is accept God's love. It's that easy."

He is silent for a moment as we sit there in the dark. It's a clear night, the moonlight shines bright on our faces, our shadows spread over the ground in front of us. Insects chirp anonymously, men shuffle past us in the dark.

Finally, he speaks. "So…you don't think it's too late for me, sir?"

"It's never too late, never," I reply.

Corporal Rosales completed his deployment unharmed.

CHAPTER 15

Operation Silent Switch, June 7th, 2004 (+174)

Throughout the deployment our battalion worked closely with the Iraqi police, training them and conducting joint missions during offensive operations. This is in preparation for when Iraqis will eventually take over security enforcement of their cities and ultimately their country. It is an extremely time-consuming, frustrating, and difficult task for the marines. There are only a few Iraqis with meaningful experience in law enforcement, and those who have the training use unorthodox techniques, tactics, and procedures. They are ill equipped and underpaid, making retention extremely precarious. All these problems are inherited by the marines. Throw in cultural and language barriers, and it becomes a slow and endless dance of two steps forward, one step back progress. Despite this, our men work diligently with the Iraqis towards their sovereignty, committing money, uniforms, weapons, and hours of blood and sweat to the cause.

Corruption and thievery are rampant among the Iraqi ranks, and when caught it is important to call out and punish these individuals to deter this behavior. On June 7th, I attended a staff meeting outlining a plan to detain and prosecute five criminal individuals discovered among the Iraqi police. Our battalion commander plans to arrest and parade them in front of fellow Iraqi police members, sending a message that corruption will not be tolerated. The plan is to take a team of marines to the Iraqi police station in Al-Garma during what should be a routine payday for the Iraqis. I will join the mission with five corpsmen to perform brief medical exams for each Iraqi officer as a gesture of good will and as a diversion tactic. After the corrupt members are paid and complete their medical exam, they will be placed in handcuffs and escorted in front of all other policemen, sending a message that corruption will be dealt with seriously. The remaining Iraqi police will be paid promptly and thanked for their service. This mission is named "Operation Silent Switch."

Our battalion lawyer is Captain Jamie McCall. Among many non-traditional duties you might expect of a lawyer, his job is to pay the Iraqi police. For the Al-Garma mission, he will take thousands of dollars in cash to pay each member of the Iraqi police. After learning about the medical role in the operation, I suspect we will be working closely together. Jamie and I first met in Okinawa before leaving for Iraq, and over the past couple months we became fast friends. He attended law school at Penn and shortly after joined the Marine Corps. I saw a lot of myself in him, his passion for life and commitment to duty as a Marine Corps officer inspired me. We bonded quickly, in part because we both chose professions sometimes perceived by society as those of opportunity, yet we found ourselves amidst war, executing our vocations in a capacity we never truly imagined. During deployment, we killed time in the gym tent or jogging around the base, discussing our lives as young men, debating politics, and dreaming of the life awaiting us upon return to the states. In the evenings we played ping-pong, watched movies on a laptop, or hunkered down with Cormac and the chaplain for a competitive game of spades or Scrabble.

Mid-deployment, Jamie developed an infected cyst in an unfortunate region requiring minor surgery. It was this event that propelled our friendship closer than either of us ever intended! In a second medical mishap, Jamie headbutted an air conditioning unit; he laughed it off with grace as I closed his scalp with seven sutures.

It's Saturday, we're 174 days into the deployment, and Operation Silent Switch is a go. In the back of my head, I'm telling myself, *"Don't do anything stupid; you're on the home stretch."* Captain McCall walks in the BAS with a friendly greeting and reminder of the fun and adventure we will have spending the day in Al-Garma. I assemble a crew of five corpsmen, and we pack a few medical bags for basic exams, mostly for show as a diversion tactic.

Jamie and I hop in the back of a Humvee, and our convoy heads out at 8:00 a.m. It's already getting hot, at least ninety degrees, and I suspect we're in for a long day of travel. Per protocol, we stop just outside the gate, exit the vehicles, and load our weapons. Facing away from the Humvee, I insert a clip into my nine-millimeter pistol, pull back, and release the slide, chambering one round. I flick the safety up and I'm ready to go. The convoy lurches forward together, turning west onto the main highway for a short distance, then exiting on an unmarked dirt road I only half-recognize from a previous convoy.

Our routes constantly change, using back roads and making our own paths to avoid predictability, ambushes, and IED attacks. I tuck a bit of chewing tobacco in my lower lip for the road trip and peer out the window at the barren desert terrain that distracts me from our destination. Before Iraq, this habit was something I reserved for hunting trips and "male bonding" with my brothers; Iraq brought back the indulgence, since nearly every other marine carries chewing tobacco in his front pocket.

We bump along the dusty roads, passing muddy, sewage-filled canals. Three weeks ago, one of our marines drowned in this canal. While swimming across to span an electrical conduit, his feet became entangled in weeds and rescue attempts failed. On dirt roads, we travel through miles of crops and fields inhabited by the occasional farmer. Small farm towns punctuate the long stretches, most of them poorly constructed clay huts or rock structures, with dirt-caked walls. Children run in the streets, waving to us as we thunder by. I marvel at their acclimation to the war all around them and the fragility of their daily life. Marines wave back, throwing soccer balls and other trinkets brought just for this occasion.

We arrive in Al-Garma before noon, linking up with Bravo Company marines stationed across from the Iraqi police station. They live in a large open bay structure with an aluminum metal roof and block wall perimeter. I enter the building headquarters and see to my left a few folding tables with laptop computers, maps, and field telephones. The remaining open bay is filled with a maze of sandbags, field gear, ammunition, and green mesh cots with silver aluminum legs. The latrine is just outside the main entrance, consisting of a dirt hole and boxes. Overheated from the journey, we unload our gear, wrestle off our helmets and flak jackets, and grab some water. Jamie and I sit side by side in metal folding chairs waiting to hear when to depart to the police station. We open magazines to pass the time. Jamie picks up a copy of *Field and Stream*, pointing at a large fish he fondly describes a prior catch, and I share in the spirit with my plans for an elk hunt in October with my dad and brothers.

KA, KA, KA-BOOM, BOOM, BOOM! We're violently jerked back to reality when multiple mortars crush the ground outside. I lurch forward to reach for my helmet at my feet. As I strap it to my chin, three more rounds pummel the earth, closer than the last. *BOOM, BOOM!* I search frantically for my flak jacket as others race for cover, but it's not where I set it down. Bodies rush past me on all sides. Frustrated, I scramble to crouch against the wall as the impacts continue. They cease a few moments later, but I remain still, heart pumping and lungs heaving with adrenaline. After a minute, I tentatively stand up to look around. No one seems to be hurt, and there are no direct hits on the building. I look over at Jamie. We both sigh with the same air of exasperation, as if to say, "*Same story, different day.*" I walk over and jokingly thank him for inviting me to such a memorable outing.

Twenty minutes later, we load up the vehicles with our gear. We head across the street to the Iraqi police station. Once there, we enter a building where the marines have gathered a couple hundred policemen. Once lined up, the herding of bodies begins. I'm positioned in a small dirty back room with two corpsmen and an interpreter. As each Iraqi comes in, the interpreter asks if he has any medical problems or takes any medications. My corpsmen document the answers, then check his blood pressure and pulse while I listen to his heart and lungs. The first five men are the policemen suspected of corruption, and as they exit the room, they are arrested and placed in handcuffs.

Despite the meaningless nature of the remaining medical exams, we continue the same process for every single Iraqi as a gesture of goodwill and an effort to support them. Most of them do not speak any English, but their faces and thankful expressions are understood. It is tedious, dirty, and hot and I'm anxious to head back to Camp Mercury upon conclusion. Our unit musters outside the compound, facing a formation of Iraqi police officers. The corrupt officers are escorted in front of the other Iraqis as a commander explains why these men have been arrested and that this fate will follow anyone participating in this kind of behavior.

I meet Captain McCall outside the compound, where we gather our gear and saunter back to the Humvees, sharing frustrations and triumphs alike. Despite the mortar attack, it's a successful and motivating operation. We load up the convoy and head for home. Our armored convoy drives, bounces, and bumps along highways, back roads, and no roads; some of it is familiar to me, while much is different from the way we came. I catch glimpses of abstract shapes, shacks, and shadows in the distance—a dead animal, an abandoned hut, a goat herder—all of it feeling suspended in time. The success of the day and journey back to the base have me feeling a pull towards home so powerful it feels as if my return is in the near future. The convoy rumbles on, leaving massive dust clouds in its trail. As we pass the outer limits of our base, two stout marines coated in white powder dust wave us through. I feel the tension in my head decompress and the nerves in my chest unwind; we are at home base once again.

CHAPTER 16

Peace in Paradise, June 8th, 2004 (+ 175)

We have less than one month to go. I find it becoming more difficult to stay motivated as we exceed one hundred and seventy-five days of deployment. The thought of home lifts my spirits, yet the minutes tick by slowly. When I'm on base, I do everything possible to keep myself busy. I have a daily routine, each task designed to eat up time and keep me moving towards the finish line. Sick call hours start each morning at 8:00 a.m. Anyone needing medical attention can show up, beyond this, marines can stop by at all hours of day or night for urgent needs. Jamie, Cormac, and I jog or lift weights almost every morning, sometimes twice in the evening after the blazing heat calms down.

The chow hall has routine dining hours for breakfast, lunch, and dinner, and assuming the supply convoy can pick up food on time, I never miss a meal. Some nights, when food is unavailable, we dine on tray rations, pre-packaged vats of food with an extended shelf life that simply need to be heated and served family style. These trays of food are dense, preserved, and hard to digest, and one of the few meals I consider skipping. Between meals, we have meetings to attend, reports to file, gear to clean, and trips to the shower trailer. Rearranging and cleaning my room can kill a good hour and checking emails is always a treat. When I miss the laundry truck, I scrub my clothes in a bucket and dry them on a line, at least a two-hour event. I read books and even stay current on the latest medical literature, all in the name of passing time.

The demands of deployment life afflict all of us, but some men suffer more than others. As monotony takes its toll, the threshold for conflict is lowered; anger, depression, and altercations become common among the men. On average, I see a marine every two to three weeks for these issues. Most of it passes with the setting sun and a new day, but for some, the deployment takes its toll and extra attention is required. Not only is it important to keep a strong fighting force during battle, it's also essential outside of combat to maintain morale. It's the daily grind that wears you down; every day is a work day, there are no weekends, you sleep in close quarters, sometimes on the ground, with irregular meals and showers, and oh, the relentless heat—it greets you at dawn and tucks you in at night.

Movement is always confined; on Camp Mercury you're limited to four block walls surrounding the camp, and while in the field you're never more than an arm's length from your platoon buddy. Always on the alert and always guarded is the only mode of operation because your life depends on it. Do this for over 200 days straight and you feel the burn. The key is to expect it and fight it—get sleep when you can, take a hot shower and eat a good meal when it's there, spend time with your friends, talk about what you miss, the things you love, knowing you'll have it back again. Force positivity and hope, it's the only way to survive.

On June 8th, I have a follow up appointment with one of the corpsmen I've counseled on and off the last three weeks. His name is HN Gauge, and he is a good corpsman but has gotten himself into trouble lately having several verbal altercations with his peers. Recently he had a breakdown and admitted to suicidal thoughts, so I had to medevac him for evaluation and treatment for combat stress. Today, he returned to Camp Mercury and has requested to give me an update on his condition.

We start the conversation by talking more about his childhood and family life. He confides he had a rough home life beginning at an early age. His father was an alcoholic and scarcely involved in his life. He doesn't mention a history of abuse, but I suspect it was present in one form or another. He cannot recall anything positive about the man and says his father was completely gone from his memory by age seven or eight. At age nine, his mother died of a stroke and he was placed in foster care. Throughout his adolescence and teens, he bounced through six different foster families for a slew of reasons, some related to interpersonal issues, others from inherent problems with the foster care system. Immediately after high school, he joined the Navy in hopes of finding a better home and career. Although he has created some problems among the men recently, I can't help feeling sympathy for this young man who has encountered so many obstacles in his life and now suffers the consequences of a lack of basic life skills.

Sanders tells me he is unsure of his long-term future in the Navy, but that he does believe it's a good place for him while finding his way in the world. He admits the three days with the combat stress team allowed him to vent frustrations and realize his errors. He has a better perspective and takes ownership of his problems and tells me he is motivated to do better. We talk about his future in the Navy, I help him with basic strategy to finish out the deployment in good fashion, and with sincerity he commits to try harder. We also discuss his religious beliefs and talk about how this could help him both now and in the future. He expresses an interest in exploring his faith and attends our bible studies over the next few weeks.

That night I climb into my rack feeling satisfied and content about the day. It's 11:00 p.m. Eyes closed and foam plugs snug in my ears, I slump down in my bag, shutting off the outside world. Not more than ten minutes pass before one of my corpsmen knocks on my door. He says the battalion commander needs me outside the Command Operations Center but can't tell me why. I put on my cammies, grab my M9 pistol and flashlight, and head towards the COC with one of my corpsmen. It's pitch-black as I travel; I need the blue light from my flashlight to find my way. Walking awkwardly through the large rock gravel, I'm wondering what's going on this late at night. As I get closer, I see a few Humvees parked in front, dusky air outlines the beams of their headlights. Fifteen to twenty Marines mingle around the vehicles looking excited about something in the back of one of the trucks. I walk towards the focus of attention and notice the battalion commander motioning me to come over to him. He is standing at the back of the Humvee.

"Hello sir, what can I do for you?" I say.

He motions towards the back of the truck and says, "Doc, we have three insurgents in the back of this Humvee. Two appear dead, and one is alive but wounded. I need you to confirm the two who are dead and check out the wounds on the third one."

My eyes shift to the back of the truck, focusing on the shadowy outline of human bodies lying in the bed. "Yes sir," I reply, still taking in the whole scene. I ask my corpsman to give me a stethoscope and latex gloves.

"Sir, how were they killed?" I ask.

"Bravo Company got into a gun fight in Al Garma, and these are some of the enemy combatants," he replies.

I put my gloves on, sling my stethoscope around my neck, and climb over the tailgate of the Humvee. Instantly, a horrible smell of body odor, dirt, and blood hits my nose. I try to breathe only through my mouth to avoid becoming sickened. I swing my light towards the three bodies, illuminating two Iraqi men lying in the fetal position in the bed of the truck and another lying face-up with hands bound and eyes fixed on me. He is a young Iraqi male in his early twenties wearing a dirty, striped collared t-shirt and brown corduroy pants. His clothes are torn and his face smeared with dirt. He is lying on his side, legs flexed towards his chest and hands tied behind his back with a zip tie. I keep one eye on him as I turn my attention to the other two motionless bodies.

They are also young Arab men, dressed in similar clothing and equally as filthy. I straddle the first body lying parallel to the insurgent who is still alive, placing my stethoscope on his chest. I hear nothing, no heartbeat and no breath sounds. Next, I lift his upper eyelids with my left hand and shine my light into his eyes with my right hand. His pupils are dilated without constriction to my light. I turn my head to the back of the truck where the battalion commander and other officers await my announcement.

"He's dead," I say.

The next man is lying perpendicular to the others towards the front. It's difficult positioning myself in the cramped and small bed of the truck. Feeling the strain standing over these bodies, I want to finish my job quickly. I examine the third man and find multiple gunshot wounds, no signs of life, and again announce he is dead.

Finally, I move back to the first insurgent to assess his wounds. As I position myself over him, he says something in Arabic. Our interpreter tells me he says he has pain in his right leg. Looking at his leg, I see a bullet entrance wound in the right upper thigh and an exit wound through the back of the leg. Corresponding blood stains on his corduroy pants confirm the trajectory.

There are no signs of active bleeding, and he appears to be in stable condition. From the side of the vehicle, one of the Marine staff sergeants tells me he is concerned that his wrists are bound too tightly and asks me to please inspect the zip ties. As I move towards him, I overhear other marines that disagree with his concerns. Regardless, I slip my finger underneath the plastic tie to check his pulse; it's rapid but strong, with good blood flow. I tell the battalion commander that according to my examination, his wrists and zip ties are fine. He nods his approval and orders the conclusion of my services. I climb out of the truck, relieved to be finished with my duties. From here, the dead insurgents are taken to the morgue, while the one who survived is taken for medical care and processing at the detention center.

I walk back to my room with mixed emotions about the events unfolding that night. Bravo Company fought fiercely, bravely, honorably in the city of Al-Garma, scoring a victory without casualties. They captured a wounded insurgent who will prove invaluable for interrogation. I have walked among dead men in the back of a truck, examining their lifeless bodies, listening to their silent hearts and breathless lungs. Now I find myself in a confusing dilemma, battling emotions about my experience with these men. I feel anger, apprehension, disgust, sorrow, and pity. I am trained to be a healer, with an oath to "do no harm." Now I'm at war with the best fighting force in the world, as a medical non-combatant, but I carry a weapon, and I'll use it if I need to. These Iraqi insurgents are the sworn enemy and have inflicted terrible violence. In an instant now, they are the subjects of that violence, lying dead in the back of a truck. Walking among their bodies, I see and feel their dehumanization, and I am unlinking them from the living world as I pronounce them dead. It's an unintentional action—more of a survival mechanism—to help me navigate the horror of it all. Tonight, I may see them in my sleep, and even feel pity for their tormented lost souls. I tell myself that it's okay, because I'm human. I'm a doctor. I'm a spiritual warrior and I need to keep my heart from entering a black hole. No matter how much I despise what they stand for, witnessing the destruction of these men is a humbling and morbid part of war I could never prepare for, and now I am crawling, stumbling, and learning to walk my way through it.

CHAPTER 17

Leaving Fallujah,
July 10th, 2004 (+ 207)

In early July, the battalion assembles and departs Camp Mercury, transferring to Camp Fallujah three miles away. This is our home for the next two weeks as we await yet another convoy to an air base, where we will catch a flight on a C-130 out of Iraq down to Kuwait. From Kuwait, we will take a commercial airliner home. Our temporary lodging at Camp Fallujah consists of huge, open-floor canvas tents assembled on top of plywood. Essentially, a tent city is erected in an open moondust field, the kind of powdered sugar dirt that clings to your tongue and dimples on the ground under a bead of sweat. With cots and bunkbeds for thirty men per tent and four feet between each bed, you are sure to become well-acquainted with the habits of your neighbor. The tents are tied down with metal stakes and thick ropes and the door flaps are secured with pulleys and water bottles to withstand the vicious winds. Despite our best efforts, the flaps shake violently in the sandstorms, and dust constantly pours into the tent.

Our tents are not directly in harm's way, but we still worry about our exposure to mortars and rockets in the open desert. Without time to build cement or dirt barriers before we arrive, one precise hit on a tent full of men could be devastating. I'm reminded that only three days after our battalion arrived at Camp Mercury in March, there was an Army surgeon killed here at Camp Fallujah not far from where our tents now stand. I remember the explosions hitting Camp Fallujah from our base at Camp Mercury; soft, chilling thuds of mortars echoed sinisterly that night, like an eerie welcome to our new home. Shortly after the attack, the radio inside the BAS informed us a soldier had been killed, and that it was the Army doctor, instantly killed by a mortar as he stepped outside his medical facility for fresh air. Later, I learned he was slated to leave for home in just three days.

Each tent has a few air conditioning units placed inside, trickling in cold air, at best creating tolerable but tepid conditions. By mid-morning, well before the sun is peaking in the sky, it is uncomfortably hot in the tents. Despite this, we spend most of the day inside the tents to avoid the oppressive heat outside. Light sweat endlessly coats our bodies. Green shorts and sandals are the standard dress. We read books, play games, and watch movies—anything to pass the hours. Begrudgingly, we often walk a half-mile in the blistering heat to the gym tent to lift weights, run on the treadmill, and enjoy better air conditioning. At mealtime, we don our uniforms and hoof it nearly a mile to the chow hall, often lingering here for over an hour watching television and enjoying the best air conditioning on the entire base. Beyond these activities, there is nothing to do but wait painfully for the word when we will leave; it is all I can think about.

Five days into our stay at Camp Fallujah, I contract the worst case of gastroenteritis (diarrhea) I've ever had. I spent three tormented nights running one hundred yards in pure darkness, tromping through powdery dirt from my tent to the ninety-degree portable outhouse. Regrettably, one night I don't make it all the way; I tell no one, and my underwear are still buried in that desert. After two days lying in my rack inside our hot tents, I am so miserable I let Captain McCall convince me to go to the gym tent with him. This foolish plan of mine results in me nearly passing out at the gym, I end up in the medical aid station with intravenous fluids and medication. To this day, I have not lost an appreciation for porcelain toilets.

Fourteen days pass at Camp Fallujah and we receive orders to pack up and convoy to an air base called Al Taqaddum. We will leave at midnight; our convoy route will take us along the outskirts of Fallujah, then west towards the air base. Estimated travel time is three to four hours, plus additional time for weather, repairs, IEDs, route changes, and any other delays involved when transporting nine hundred men and all their combat gear by ground.

By midnight, all our gear is loaded and a train of seven-ton trucks is lined in front of our tents with headlights blazing. The engines roar to life, telling us it's time to go. Green flashlights and blue headlamps flicker in the dark, and we can feel the energy in the air. We gather outside in front of the trucks for a final convoy briefing, including basic information about our route, expected obstacles, common communication pitfalls, and protocols in case we were engaged by small arms, mortars, or an IED attack. Each man is assigned to a truck, then dismissed to load up. I'm assigned to one of the open air seven-ton trucks. Tossing my pack on board, I climb up and over the green steel tailgate and take my seat on the wooden bench. I strap on my Kevlar helmet, adjust my flak jacket, and settle in for a long, bumpy ride. I'm happy to see Captain Jamie Edge sitting next to me; we exchange a handshake as the truck groans into motion and suspension sways side to side as we pass the vacant tent city.

Jamie is our combat operations officer, and one of the more passionate, animated officers in the battalion. He is striking to look at, fitting the Marine Corps officer prototype dead on. He is six feet, four inches tall, with a medium build and a prominent jawline framing his face. He has a stern appearance but genuine and pleasant affect. He has a classic horseshoe buzz cut that exemplifies his love for the Marine Corps, and he often draws comments from his fellow officers regarding his motivated facade. Put together, he is intimidating if you don't know him, but entertaining and warm once he is your friend.

I met Jamie in July of 2003 when I was brand new to the battalion. He was among the first to make an impression on me. It was not that he went out of his way to be friendly, but rather that he treated me like one of the other Marine Corps officers, straight forward and fair, despite the fact I was a Navy officer. In the months prior to our deployment, we became quick friends, and although our interactions were usually brief, he was one of my favorite people to run into. I could always count on him for a quick laugh or random topic *du jour* of his choosing. Jamie and I both had identical twin brothers, sharing the bond of understanding the special brotherhood that exists among twins. He loved rambling about the nuances of life in the Marine Corps, military history, and politics of the world. He loved throwing odd medical questions at me, keeping me on my toes, and musing at my answers. Our debates sometimes elevated to serious discussions, but in the next moment we would joke about nothing again.

As we rumble down the road, warm night air blows in my face and I tighten my ballistic goggles to keep the dust out of my eyes. After winding through the dirt and the gravel backroads, we lurch onto a main highway. In the distance, I see the lights of a city; Jamie leans over to me, pointing with his finger. "Fallujah," he says.

I slouch a bit lower on the bench and check the position of my M9 pistol strapped to the left side of my chest. Our train of trucks pitches and heaves along the road without headlights, like a snake in the dark, making as little commotion as possible. I sit on the bench keeping a cautious eye towards Fallujah. Driving by the city is just enough to keep me on edge, making me reluctant to let down my guard. Jamie reaches into his cammies for a tin of tobacco and offers it to me. I accept his offer, grabbing a pinch to tuck into my lower lip.

The convoy treks along the outskirts of Fallujah in the blackness of night, and I feel good knowing we are leaving it behind, enjoying the taste of the tobacco. The violence that filled the streets not long ago is fresh in my mind; thousands of bullets and hundreds of bombs were dropped, changing countless lives forever. Either stubbornly or inadvertently, casualties of war included both innocent and wicked men and women. At times, it was straightforward, good guys versus bad guys. Yet on the other hand, it was deeply complex and none of it fit neatly together. Men of First Battalion, Fifth Marines were wounded both physically and mentally, changing them forever—I too am changed forever. In the end, there are many unanswered questions and no easy answers. What is certain to me as I sit in the back of the seven-ton truck is that everyone I worked with, from beginning to end, conducted themselves with the utmost dedication and perseverance to their jobs. Our battalion is a unique merger of men and minds, thrown into impossible situations, achieving victory on many fronts, and my heart swells with pride to be a part of it.

As we edge along the outskirts of Fallujah, I am relieved to be leaving it all behind, one step closer to home, but it's still not close enough. Jamie tells me about his family at home, his wife Krissy and his two little girls. I tell him about Katie and the plans for our wedding when we get back (keeping our elopement in Vegas a secret).

We talk about arrival home and the very first things we will do: drink an ice-cold beer and take a trip to the beach. We talk about our favorite bands, debating the best live concerts we've ever attended. We are both big fans of Pearl Jam, and before we know it, we are singing our favorite songs together, just loud enough to hear each other over the whining of the tires and the wind swirling around our heads. It's a moment of bonding, the kind I want to remember long after it's gone.

Jamie and I talk for hours while hot wind whips at our faces and dust thickens until we have to cover our mouths and noses with handkerchiefs tied around our heads. The convoy stops numerous times as weather deteriorates, and navigation is difficult. Despite the late hour, it is dreadfully hot, and my sweaty uniform sticks to my back. Our water supply is uncomfortably warm, making it difficult to maintain hydration. Trying to escape the storm, I lie flat in the truck bed. Awkward and uncomfortable, I retreat to sitting upright with my back to the wind.

After seven hours, double the expected time, we make it to Al Taqaddum air base as the morning sun begins its trek across the sky. I hop off the truck feeling tired but relieved. Our gear is piled heavy and deep in the seven-ton truck, overflowing with straps, clips, and field gear. I sift through the mess and haul mine to safety. I'm dirty and exhausted, in dire need of a shower. Instead, I promptly tow my gear to a tent, heave my sea bags and pack on the floor, and fall asleep for hours.

CHAPTER 18

Reunion, July 15th, 2004 (+ 212)

The Battalion remains at Al Taqaddum air base for the next four days. Finally, word comes down the chain: we're booked on the next C-130 flight to Kuwait. These Air Force planes are large, open-belly transport vessels used extensively in Iraq for hauling military personnel and their gear long distances. The interior looks like a commercial airliner with all the innards removed except for essential wires, fuel lines, and steel infrastructure. The center aisles are lined with nylon jump seats, placing you snugly close to the person next to you while facing another person in front of you. Ear protection is essential to protect you from the roar of four massive propeller engines mounted on the wings; combine this with a heavy flak jacket, Kevlar helmet, field gear, and 115 degree temperatures, and you're ready for a memorable flight.

We touchdown in Kuwait midafternoon. Heat radiates off the pavement as we parade off the tarmac into formation and march herded into a giant hanger filled with cots and coffee. Here, we'll wait to board a commercial airliner headed for home. U.S. soil is just hours away, but until I leave the Middle East, my heart is still in the desert. Again, I pass the hours lying on my cot, sleeping, reading, and talking to anyone about anything to keep my mind occupied. I lie staring upward in the hanger, dreaming of my reunion with Katie and my family at Camp Pendleton, sometimes so intensely it brings tears to my eyes, tears I quickly whisk away for fear of onlookers. Amidst my dreams of home, quiet voices in the back of the hanger discuss funeral plans for the men who will not make it home. Twenty-four hours pass, our plane arrives, and we're advised we will be loading shortly. I only carry a light day pack filled with a change of clothes, books, iPod, and food for the trip home. Wearing my desert camouflage uniform and carrying my nine-millimeter pistol, I don't appear to be boarding a commercial airliner. Until we're out of combat territory, all the marines and sailors keep their weapons on their person.

First Sergeant Coleman from Charlie Company calls us to attention, then as we have done hundreds of times before, we march in a single file line towards our objective, a beautiful United 747 double-decker airliner, ready to gobble us up and take us home. I'll never forget the oddity of our scene: hundreds of men toting weapons onto this plush airplane, jesting back and forth with high spirits and big smiles like college kids on spring break. All the stewardesses are dressed in red, white, and blue and have decorated the airplane with patriotic fanfare. As I ease down into my cushioned oversized seat, a sense of calm comes over me, like warm water across my back. I'm feeling a sense of peace I lost many months ago. The waiting and wondering are over; I know we are going home, and for the first time in many months a feeling of serenity enters my heart.

Twenty hours later, we touch down at March Air Force Base, California, the same airbase we departed from seven months earlier. As we taxi in, I see three bright red fire trucks on the tarmac, sirens blasting and rainbows of water spraying from their tanks. This continues for thirty minutes. My heart swells with pride as we walk down the steps of the plane, greeting a small but hearty reunion team staged for us with drinks and food. Once our sea bags are unloaded and accounted for, we load the whitewashed buses for the three-hour trip to Camp Pendleton.

It's late afternoon when we arrive, the bus is humid and cramped, and we are all very anxious to get off as quickly as possible. But before we can see our families, we have to make one more stop by the ammo depot to turn in our weapons and ammunition. This takes an hour, then we're on our way again, heading to the reunion site on base where our families wait for us.

Fifteen minutes later, we pull in five hundred yards away from the reunion area. We unload the buses, gather into formation, and start marching towards the sound of fanfare. As we march, the anticipation grows. I can't see the crowd, but I sense there is a large number of people gathered ahead of us. As the formation rounds the corner, I see the streets lined with hundreds of cheering fans of all ages; heads in the crowd bob up and down, searching for their hero marching in.

My heart speeds up as I scan for a familiar face. We keep marching closer. My eyes catch sight of my father on the right side of the street—he is standing among the crowd. He doesn't see me at first; his head is raised and earnestly searching the faces of our formation. Without thinking, and before the command is given to halt, I break ranks and run to my dad while calling his name.

We hug and cry. "It's so good to be home, Dad," I say. The men behind me keep marching, then others start running to their families.

I'm at a loss for words, all I can get out is, "Dad, take me to Katie."

"Okay Donnelly, she's over here," he replies.

I follow him through a small group of people to where I see her standing by herself looking through the crowds. I call her name and she turns in my direction. She has on a red sleeveless blouse and a white skirt; her hair is long, wavy, and dark. Dropping my ruck sack, I pick up the pace as I move toward her. We embrace, exchanging long-absent words of affection, talking over each other as we sway. Overcome with emotion, I press my cheek to hers telling her I am finally home and she is the best thing I have ever seen. I tell her it's been so hard being gone and I will never leave her again. Little do we know, we will have to do it all over again in a few years. I still have the photograph of this day, one that I will never forget.

Cheers, music, hugs, and laughter continue all around, and I look up from where Katie and I stand to see twenty more family members holding a sign that reads "Welcome Home Donnelly, We Love You." They stand together in a half circle, clapping and cheering, just as hundreds of other families are doing the same for their loved ones. I had no idea that so many of them made the long trip to Camp Pendleton, waiting all day for me to arrive. It is an overwhelming show of love and support, one of the best moments of my life.

CHAPTER 19

A Farewell to Arms, August 2004

It's August and most of us are settled into a home routine again. Work, dining out, and time with family are the norm. Fall is on the way and the dry coastal hills of Camp Pendleton call for rain. The season is begging to change, but for many of the men of First Battalion, Fifth Marines, our hearts and minds still linger in the past; each one of us is still healing, coping, and filling the space of what was lost in Iraq.

Sadly, my deployment to Fallujah was a turning point in my parents' relationship. Progressive disconnect over their thirty-five years of marriage has taken its toll, and they are starting to unravel. Within one year of my return, they separate, and our family is forever changed. In our small town, my parents had many social circles, and for better or worse some idealized us as the model American family: five boys, all athletes, strong students, and solid parents. I felt my idyllic roots being torn apart and it hurt deeply to know our family history would never be the same. I even tried to coach my father back to her, but to no avail. His harsh ways had created too many wounds to heal, too many words that couldn't be taken back, and now she was gone.

We take time to adjust, heal wounds, and change habits that were formed out of the need to endure. For Katie and I, the first three months home are filled with one event after the next. While I was in Iraq, she spent much of her time planning our new life together, painting the inside of our home, working at CBS Sports, and finalizing our wedding day on September 18th, 2004. Although we will have been married for almost a year, we still decided to keep it secret. To all our friends and family, this will be our actual wedding day.

Amidst all of this change and planning, we renew friendships, take vacations, and attend ceremonial events, which bring both pain and closure to our deployment. For the marines and sailors of First Battalion, Fifth Marines, this culminates in a funeral for the men who never made it home.

It's a Sunday morning like many others, but on this day the community church in Oceanside, just outside Camp Pendleton, is filled with nine hundred men in uniform—battle dress uniforms. The same ones we wore in Iraq, the same desert brown fatigues and well-worn boots that defined our journey. We file into the church quietly, taking our seats among familiar faces, feeling the common bonds. Battalion flags with stars and stripes adorn the alter and flowers decorate their bases. Our hearts are heavy with anticipation of the theme at hand, a final goodbye to the men who gave their lives in combat. Distinguished and honored guests are seated in the front pews; these are the family and close friends of those killed in action. My chest swells with emotion as I sit in the hard wooden pew, looking on with reverence and waiting for the ceremony to begin.

Colonel Byrne, our battalion commander, opens the ceremony. Each man is described as honorable, courageous, and committed, yet all present know words alone can never yield the sum of what these men represent. Then the chaplain speaks; words of sadness, comfort, and God's peace ring throughout the church. A sigh breaks from the crowd, a tear runs down a cheek. Then a single marine stands up in front of the altar and faces the crowd. He holds a list of ten names; these are the men lost from First Battalion, Fifth Marines. With an unmistakable Marine Corps pitch and tenor, a roll call commences. The name and rank of each man is called out aloud from the list, his words echo throughout the pews, into the ceiling, and up the stairs onto the balcony seating. A few seconds pass, there is no response from anyone in the crowd or on the alter, only silence. The name is read out loud again, clear and strong, as if the first roll call has not been heard. Silence persists, and a third time the vacant marine's name is called. This time, the audience is now certain of the outcome—no answer. For ten names, the process is repeated and the void in response painfully understood by the audience. For the men who never came home, this is their final roll call.

From time to time people ask me, "Donnelly, why did you do it? Why did you become a Navy doctor, then go to war?" It's a difficult question to answer. The path to Fallujah was years in the making. Part of it was in my control, part of it wasn't. Aspirations, life events, and emotions along the way weighed heavy on my choices, and rarely was there a singular deciding factor at each interval. The decisions have always included elements of service, patriotism, and love for adventure. But when pressed—"Really, Donnelly, why did you do it?"—I'm driven to one answer: I did it because I could. I did it because I had the determination, I had the skills, and I had the courage. In short,

I had the tools to attempt something great, so I did it. If you ask me how I got those tools, I'll tell you by meeting God halfway and accepting His grace. He opened the doors, and I walked through.

A BROTHER FALLS

After my return to Camp Pendleton, I remained with First Battalion, Fifth Marines for two months, taking leave and completing post-deployment medical evaluations for all the men in our battalion. Then, as often occurs following deployments, men are transferred within the battalion.

New recruits are indoctrinated, senior enlisted men retire, and others transfer in or out of the battalion and on to new assignments. I transfer to First Combat Engineers Battalion, located directly next to my former aid station with 1/5. In the months that follow, I rarely see Jamie Edge and the other officers of my old battalion, but their spirit remains with me long after I depart. Captain Edge remains with 1/5, and not more than two months after we return home, he is slated for their next deployment to Iraq; six months of training immediately ensues. On occasion, I run into Jamie at battalion headquarters or amid training sessions, and he's always in the best of spirits despite their rapid deployment cycle and the hardships it bestows upon him and his family. Not only is he optimistic, but he genuinely seems excited. Recently he was promoted to company commander of his own unit of marines, something I know he sought for a long time. It's no surprise to hear how well he commands the respect of his men; he is in his true element and will lead them into combat.

Six months pass. It's a crisp spring morning at Camp Pendleton, the day Captain Edge and 1/5 are scheduled to leave again for Iraq.

Wildflowers bloom in the hills surrounding Camp Pendleton, and the smell of sagebrush frequently drifts into my workspace. I'm in my office, down the street from the parade deck where the buses are staged, unaware D-Day has come once again.

Early that morning, something unordinary stirred, a commotion in the air that suggested men were in motion. *"What's going on?"* I pondered sitting at my desk. Perhaps there was an honored guest on site or a valorous medal being awarded? No wait—*"Could it be a deployment underway?"* I thought.

Their departure had been on my mind all month, but it had escaped me on this day. When morning sick call ends, I immediately run to the staging area, hoping to catch Jamie and some of the other marines before they leave. Familiar rectangle shaped whitewashed buses are aligned side by side, loaded and ready to go. High and tight crew cuts bob among the seats, all of the men dressed in stark new uniforms. Eager faces peer out from the glass windows as the bus engines roar to life. I scan the masses of desert camouflaged men for familiar faces, finding Jamie standing outside an open bus door, sharp, confident, with anticipation on his face.

I walk towards him, and as his head turns my way, a classic Jamie Edge grin spreads across his broad chin. It's been two months since we last saw each other, so we exchange a firm handshake and embrace. He's in uncommonly good spirits considering the task at hand; adapting and enduring comes naturally to him. For most of his men, their time at home was occupied with training for the next deployment. Downtime was minimal and quality time with loved ones sparse. My name has been on the chopping block for a second deployment since my return, but thus far nothing had come to fruition. I stand with Jamie talking for ten minutes, up to the last moment as final preparations are made. He tells me about his company of marines, how well prepared they are and their mission in Ramadi. We reminisce about our last deployment, all that had come and gone, and he smiles as he talks. Finally, it's time to go. We say farewell, Godspeed, Semper Fi, and I walk away. The buses rev their engines, lurch forward, and file out one by one, once again on their way east, out the back gate of Camp Pendleton, then north on Interstate 15, through Barstow, into the high desert, and on to March Air Force base. This is the last time I see Captain Jamie Edge.

One month later, I sit in my office at Camp Pendleton. It's mid-afternoon, the rolling hills are lined with green grass, and a warm ocean breeze flaps the curtains of my office window.

My senior corpsman knocks on the door, leaning in with a concerned look on his face and says, "Sir…I thought you should know…. Captain Edge was killed yesterday in Iraq. I know you were close, and I thought you should know."

I can't believe the words from his mouth. I just shook the man's hand a few weeks ago, how could Edge be gone? My heart is crushed. I'm stunned and speechless.

"*Oh Lord, what about his wife and two little girls?*" I say to myself. Later that night with my wife I cried for him and his family.

On April 14th, 2005, Captain Jamie Edge was killed in Ramadi, Iraq. The press release by the Department of Defense reads: "Captain James C. Edge, 31, of Virginia Beach, Virginia, was killed April 14, 2005, by enemy small-arms fire while conducting combat operations in Ramadi, Iraq. He was assigned to 1st Battalion, 5th Marine Regiment, 1st Marine Division, I Marine Expeditionary Force, Camp Pendleton, California. During Operation Iraqi Freedom,

Edge was attached to 2nd Marine Division, II Marine Expeditionary Force (Forward).”

In the coming months, I learn more details about the day he was killed. Captain Edge and his men came under attack while on patrol in Ramadi. The ambush was mainly small arms fire, including AK-47 machine guns, mortars, and rocket-propelled grenades. While his marines engaged the enemy, Jamie sought higher ground upon a rooftop to establish communications and coordinate air support. As he moved on the rooftop, he was killed instantly by an enemy sniper with a single gunshot to the head.

His funeral was at Arlington National Cemetery, Virginia. It was the most impressive showing of love and support for a person and his family I have ever seen. In attendance were friends, family, and military personnel of all ranks and services from all over the United States. The ceremony was given with full military honors, military regalia, and horse-drawn carriage. Although profoundly sad, the tribute to Captain Edge and his service to our country was wonderful. The Arlington Cemetery website quotes this statement from his father:

“He was a loving husband and father, devoted son and brother. He was the best of the best our country had to offer. We need to remember his sacrifice and honor his memory. He was known and loved by many people here in Hampton Roads. He leaves a legacy of fierce love of God and country, the Corps and family. His commitment to these was evident in how he lived his life.”

The impact Jamie had on me is testimony to the man he was. The connections we made through turmoil created bonds of friendship and respect uncommonly found; this is what made his departure difficult. I like to remember my friend in his best moments, as I rode with him out of Fallujah, singing our favorite songs, the spirit of service and adventure on his face during the final moments I saw him, and the simple love he had for life, no matter how it came at him. His spirit lives on in his fellow marines, the people who knew him best, and in my heart. Though it may be inadequate, I need to say this to my brother in Christ: I truly do think about you often, along with all the men of First Battalion, Fifth Marines, and we *will* meet again, wrapped in the peace of God's glory.

CHAPTER 20

The Message

At the end of my journey, I have a treasure chest to share, and I have a seminal message. Don't wait for your life to come to you. With the right training, you can do great things. Among them, these three key elements: Get your heart and mind balanced, get your body fit, grab a fist full of courage, and go after it.

But how do we successfully traverse the trial of life? What comfort can we take in our seemingly endless struggle to prepare well, to keep pace, to endure, to pull ahead, to win this amazing race through life? The answer to this question is completely realized when each one of us, in our own time, submits to the fact there is no race, only the one we create. As I've navigated the unknowns in my life, too often my sights have been focused on the finish line, believing the key to happiness was waiting at the winner's circle. My drive propelled me to higher levels, but I missed opportunities for growth along the way. Whether grinding my way through medical school, or maneuvering the perils of Fallujah, I learned there is no finish line. True peace and contentment entered my life when yielding to the fact my efforts and accolades were only part of the equation. I learned that I could beat myself up with grit and determination, but if I didn't have peace in my heart, and the good Lord on my side, I was destined to lose. The best parts of my life have been the moments within the journey itself, and not the final destination. A sunset over the French Quarter, late night rounds at Charity Hospital, the gratitude in a sick patient's eyes, a salute to the stars and stripes, the return home to my wife and family—these are the pieces that make me whole.

We are a nation born from immense sacrifice, innovation, self-reliance, and principle. It's easy to feel like God must keep tabs on our value just as we do, but God does not have a scoreboard for our lives. We may even be drawn to and take comfort in the short-lived accolades of the world. And then a moment comes when we can clearly see beyond these myopic measurements of our worth and witness God's outstretched hand, place ours in His, and realize He erases all these external gauges of merit, replacing them with His grace and love; all we have to do is say, "Yes Lord, I will take your hand."

If you have ever felt incapable of living up to an unattainable image in this life, you can take rest in these words from Paul in the bible, book of Ephesians 2:8-10:

> God saved you by his grace when you believed. And you can't take credit for this; it is a gift from God. Salvation is not a reward for the good things we have done, so none of us can boast about it. For we are God's masterpiece. He has created us anew in Christ Jesus, so that we can do the good things he planned for us long ago. (New Living Translation)

Life is not a contest, and Paul assures us, if "Salvation is not a reward for the good things we have done," then we know God is not keeping score. It is such a simple concept and a stunning showing of God's grace.

Some are struck like a lightning bolt, their hearts instantly transformed when they accept God's love, while others travel through tremendous peaks and valleys before landing upon the path to salvation. It was many years until I fully grasped what God's grace meant to me and how it could change my life, and not until the night at the cloverleaf did I wholly succumb to His life-saving grace. I fell flat on my face many times before clearly seeing the extent of His work in my life. Regardless, the path is not as important as the destination; God longs for all his children to make it to heaven, no matter how long it takes.

What then, you may ask, after we have given our hearts to Christ, do we have to assure us of his love? If we knowingly allow ourselves to fall out of the race, how do we know we won't get left behind? After all, life is riddled with unforeseen hardships, temptations, and tragedy, which undoubtedly will cause us to stumble, and doubt God's grace. What if I break my promise of faith and devotion to God? Certainly, there must be dire consequences for such treachery, there must be some threshold of no return if we should dare to cross it. There are no words I can summon to better describe the answer to this question than what Paul wrote to the Romans, in the book of Romans 8:35-39:

> Can anything ever separate us from Christ's love? Does it
> mean he no longer loves us if we have trouble or calamity, or
> are persecuted, or are hungry or cold or in danger or threat-

ened with death? (As the Scriptures say, "For your sake we are killed every day; we are being slaughtered like sheep.") No, despite all these things, overwhelming victory is ours through Christ, who loved us.

And I am convinced that nothing can ever separate us from his love. Death can't, and life can't. The angels can't, and the demons can't. Our fears for today, our worries about tomorrow, and even the powers of hell can't keep God's love away. Whether we are high above the sky or in the deepest ocean, nothing in all creation will ever be able to separate us from the love of God that is revealed in Christ Jesus our Lord. (New Living Translation, 2008)

Untangling the mystery of life is the ultimate adventure. Finding peace on that journey is the ultimate challenge. The great unknowns are the forks in the road. There will be many, and they will provoke every ounce of your confidence and test the limits of your will. Ultimately, every decision is a stepping-stone placed on your path as it's forged. There will be missteps, disappointments, and regrets along the way. These are not failures. They are opportunities to learn from mistakes, recalculate your course, and find a new direction. None of this happens standing still. Don't wait for your future to come to you. Prepare yourself with three crucial actions as you train for your journey: Get your heart and mind balanced, get your body fit, grab a fistful of courage, and go after it.

Start with your heart and mind. Find God's love—release stowed anger, emotional trauma, and locked up guilt. Revive lost love, unsaid words, or silenced relationships. Look for open doors, take a chance, and walk right on through. Don't put it off any longer or wait for the other party to act—take the reins, and do it on your terms. If you need help, don't do it alone. Find people who love you, professionals you trust, and hire them to your team. When your heart is full and your mind is at peace, you're ready for uncharted waters.

Get your body fit—it's your vessel, and the most highly advanced organism in the history of the universe. Our brains can store over a million gigabytes of data, and our bodies have enough blood vessels to circle the earth four times. You can't neglect it and expect thigs to go well. Everything you need to function at peak performance is readily abundant from mother earth—use it. The best nutrients you can find come right from the ground—eat the rainbow of colors, shapes, and sizes of fruits, vegetables, beans, lentils, seeds, and nuts. Fortify your muscles and your mind with plant-based proteins and omega fats. Add wild fish, shellfish, and modest amounts of organic lean animal proteins to complete the circle. In summary, a Mediterranean style diet will accomplish all your needs. Next, put your vessel to work, then let it heal—exercise regularly, push your body to higher limits, then rest and restore with meditation, stretching, and restorative sleep. Include a combination of cardiovascular vascular fitness and strength training. Your first goal is to optimize the most vital muscle in your body—the heart. It's made of cardiac muscle and needs to be trained properly. A good starting point is thirty to sixty minutes of aerobic fitness three to four times per week. Add strength training with light weights or bands for your core and axial skeletal muscles (muscles originating from the head, neck, and vertebral column). Consult with your doctor and health professionals to develop your plan!

Finally, grab a fist full of courage and go after it. This means when you're satisfied with your preparation—and at peace that you have done your best to prepare your heart and mind, nourish your body, and optimize your fitness—now you're ready for launch. Despite this, nothing guarantees success, and the great unknowns lie ahead. You have unanswered questions, fears, and doubts. Despite all this, you're ready to face adversity, danger, and even pain, in the pursuit of triumph! That's the definition of courage. You've got it, now harness it, and unleash it.

Thank you for coming on this journey with me, and for knowing that my story is one of many, handed down only by the grace of God, and I leave you with this: When this life is done, and we have been relieved from the weight of the world, know that there is love, and only love.

SOURCES

Kevin Flower, Melissa Gray, Sue Kroll, Vivian Paulsen, and Auday Sadik, "U.S. Expects More Attacks in Iraq," CNN, May 6, 2004, https://www.cnn.com/2004/WORLD/meast/03/31/iraq.main/.

Jane Arraf, Jim Clancy, Barbara Starr, Kevin Flower, and Kianne Sadeq, "Marines, Iraqis Join Forces to Shut Down Fallujah," April 6, 2004, https://www.cnn.com/2004/WORLD/meast/04/05/iraq.main/index.html.

"Operation Vigilant Resolve," Globalsecurity.org, April 5, 2004, https://www.globalsecurity.org/military/ops/oif-vigilant-resolve.htm.

Tony Perry, Edmund Sanders, "Marines Roll Into Fallouja," Los Angeles Times, April 5, 2004, https://www.latimes.com/archives/la-xpm-2004-apr-05-fg-fallouja5-story.html.

"First Battle of Fallujah," Wikipedia, September 16, 2020, https://en.wikipedia.org/wiki/First_Battle_of_Fallujah.

Glenn Kessler, "Weapons Given to Iraq Are Missing," The Washington Post, August 6, 2007, https://www.washingtonpost.com/wp-dyn/content/article/2007/08/05/AR2007080501299_pf.html.

"Fallujah," Globalsecurity.org, October 6, 2004, http://web.archive.org/web/20041031002157/www.globalsecurity.org/military/world/iraq/fallujah.htm.

Alice Hills, "Fear and Loathing in Falluja," Sage Journals, July 1, 2006, https://journals.sagepub.com/doi/10.1177/0095327X05281460.

http://www.fallenheroesmemorial.com/oif/profiles/edgejamesc.html

McDowell, Josh, More Than a Carpenter (Illinois, Tyndale House Publishers, 2009), 50, 61, 79, 82, 83, 85, 87.

ACKNOWLEDGMENTS

Cormac O'Connor, M.D. (USN) – I could not have asked for a better Naval Officer, doctor and companion on our journey. Thank you for your friendship and dedication to your profession.

Jamie McCall, Esq (USMC) – You are a true patriot and credit to the uniform. Our lives intersected for a reason, and I'm honored to have served with you. Semper Fi my friend.

Herb Schaffner, Big Fish Media – Thank you for your faith in this work and bringing out the best in me. Your editing is top tier, and it was a true pleasure to work with you.

Jeannie Fantasia, Virtually Social Management – I greatly appreciate you coming on this ride with me. Thank you for your excellent social media and marketing skills.

Robert (Buzz) Patterson, Lt.Col., USAF (Ret.) – Thank you for your review and assistance with this work. I appreciate your mentorship.

Matthew May – I appreciate your referral at a key moment. Thank you for taking the time to make a difference.

ABOUT THE AUTHOR

Donnelly Wilkes, M.D. is a California native. He is board-certified by the American Board of Family Medicine. Dr. Wilkes obtained his bachelor's degree from the University of California, Irvine, and his medical degree from Tulane School of Medicine on a full Navy Scholarship. Following medical school, Wilkes was commissioned in the U.S. Navy, com-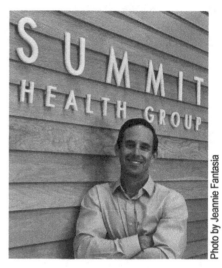pleted residency training in family medicine at the Naval Hospital Camp Pendleton, and served seven years on active duty. Wilkes served two combat tours in Iraq in 2004 and 2008 and was awarded the Navy Commendation Medal with Valor for his actions in the battle of Fallujah in April of 2004. He finished his Naval career as the Senior Medical Officer at Port Hueneme Naval Clinic, where he was responsible for the medical oversight of active duty members, their families, and local Veterans. Upon completion of his Naval service, Dr. Wilkes was honorably discharged as a Lieutenant Commander and opened Wilkes Family Medicine in August of 2009. He is now the president and medical director of Summit Health Group in Thousand Oaks, California. Dr. Wilkes is a devoted husband, father, and Christian.

Photo by Jeannie Fantasia